Stress in Hospital

Stress in Hospital
PATIENTS' PSYCHOLOGICAL REACTIONS
TO ILLNESS AND HEALTH CARE

Jenifer Wilson-Barnett
BA, MSc, PhD, SRN, Dip.N
Lecturer in Nursing Studies,
Chelsea College, University of London

CHURCHILL LIVINGSTONE
EDINBURGH LONDON AND NEW YORK 1979

CHURCHILL LIVINGSTONE
Medical Division of Longman Group Limited

Distributed in the United States of America by Longman
Inc., 19 West 44th Street, New York, N.Y. 10036, and by
associated companies, branches and representatives
throughout the world.

© Longman Group Limited 1979

First published 1979

ISBN 0 443 01879 0

British Library Cataloguing in Publication Data

Wilson-Barnett, Jenifer
  Stress in hospital.
  1. Hospital patients – Psychology
  2. Stress (Psychology)
  I. Title
  362.1'1   RA965.3   79–40166

Printed in Singapore by Kua Co., Book Manufacturer, Pte Ltd.

Preface

When preparing a new lecture course entitled 'Patients' Key Experiences' for undergraduate nurses at Chelsea College, I realised just how widely the literature was spread over several disciplines. This volume is therefore an attempt to integrate some of the research findings on this subject for the benefit of students in all the health sciences. The contents are aimed towards interesting the readers and encouraging wider exploration and questioning about psychological reactions to illness.

Research completed for my own doctoral degree on patients' emotional responses is also discussed at length. Critical appraisal of this may give students insight into the problems of researching patients' psychological reactions and hopefully initiate some ideas for solving them. Professor Jim Watson at Guy's Hospital, who supervised the project, was always willing to accept original and unusual ideas on methodology. I hope that he will accept any praise while any other comments can be directed towards the author.

It would not have been possible to write this book without the constant help and inspiration of my husband Mike Trimble. Not only did we discuss each chapter in concept but many of the most useful details and ideas are his.

Several others have helped during my work on this book. Professor Jack Hayward at Chelsea College was obviously instrumental in the creation of the lecture course and my lectureship, for which I will always be grateful.

I would also like to thank my research assistant Annie Carrigy for a wonderful year of data collection. Her hard work and intelligence contributed so much to the research reported in this text.

Lastly, I am most grateful to my typist Jane Tait for her invaluable work under far from ideal conditions!

London, 1978

J. Wilson-Barnett

To Bar and Auntie

Contents

Introduction

Many doctors and nurses still need to be convinced that psychological factors affect patients' physical recovery. They therefore tend to give psychological care a comparatively low place on their list of priorities when treating patients.

In this text, literature and research in the field of stress, reactions to illness and the interrelationship between the two will be reviewed. Evidence which indicates that stressful events are related to a deterioration in health is also included.

'Stress', of course, needs to be defined and classified. It is discussed in Chapter 1 and shown to be a notoriously broad and complex term. Various theories and research into the physiological effect of stress reactions on the body are also included to demonstrate that heightened sympathetic and other responses can lead to morbidity.

Hospitalisation, which can be seen as a classical example of a stressful event is often made more or less stressful by conversations, communications and treatment from staff to patients. Research on how patients view their hospital experience shows that they feel strongly about their dealings with the staff and are helped if staff are friendly, warm and informative. On the other hand, there is a huge mass of literature, anecdotal and research evidence, which is reviewed in several Chapters of this book, which gives accounts of how poorly patients are comforted and supported psychologically, illuminating a complete divergence of interests and goals. While patients find psychological care very important, staff often do not regard this as greatly important in relation to physical care and overall provisions for providing a service. It is imperative that someone who needs medical attention, who is thus already under the stress of illness, is not exposed to more stress which could be prevented.

There is another objective to this book. Most health care professionals have taught from experience, trial and error or wise opinion. By using systematically researched information, we are more likely to be therapeutic. A sizeable body of research into psychological reactions to illness and events related to treatment now exists. Some of this can provide useful indications for helping patients. It is no longer considered professional to adhere to customary procedures if evidence exists that they are either ineffective to therapy or unnecessarily stressful, that is, cause undue distress to the patient. In providing a brief review of this research selected from nursing, psychological and medical texts and journals it is hoped to show how research can be useful, how it can be extended in the future, and also to indicate some of the errors which should not be repeated. This review is not comprehensive, as it is mainly orientated towards adult care in general hospitals, but most of the references are obtainable from main medical or nursing libraries in the western world, and will direct readers to further work in these areas of study. It is necessary to say in advance that a few studies are criticised and this is done to provide pointers for evaluating research in this area, so that interpretations can be qualified as necessary.

This field of research has often been given a sceptical reception by clinicians. This is perhaps because it is limited to the study of patients and subject to an infinite range of personality and environmental factors. Experimentation is often ethically rejected, and aspects of care and proposals for care are frequently almost impossible to measure. However, many others feel that it is essential to adopt scientific principles in caring for the sick and, where possible, to evaluate care in terms of benefit to patients. This text, therefore, attempts to give an outline of research progress in psychological reactions to illness and health care, how they affect patients' recovery or aid resistance to illness and how the behaviour of others can in turn affect these reactions.

In concentrating on how others affect patients, the behaviour of professional staff has been studied most frequently. From a recent study (Wilson-Barnett, 1977), it seems that even in the 'best' hospitals patients can suffer psychological distress through staff neglect. Two brief case studies are included below which demonstrate that more attention and thought to this aspect of care is necessary. They have been selected from over 200 other such cases because they have previously stimulated strong reactions from professional audiences. They usually make staff ask themselves whether the same thing could occur in their own work setting and if so, what they could do to prevent them.

Case study no. 1

Mr T, a 19-year-old youth, was admitted for reassessment of disseminated sclerosis and treatment of an exacerbation of his symptoms. He lived at home with his parents, who considered he was not really ill and should be cured by a 'good day's work'. Mr T had a fairly accurate picture of his condition and its implications. He confided that he felt both anxious and depressed and so had lost most of his friends. He felt very despondent about his condition and particularly about the fact that no one talked to him about this while he was in hospital, or even acknowledged that they knew he could discuss it. Physical examinations by doctors and students annoyed him: 'they drive me mad, you feel just like a guinea pig'. He felt unhappy that he could not talk to the nurses, because they were always too busy. When he asked to go outside they told him he could not, without giving a reason for this. The hot summer weather which other patients were enjoying made him feel much worse about this. During his second week he 'did not sleep' for four nights because he was 'worried sick'. He also resigned from his job because he felt he could not cope (and his resignation was accepted). He felt as though he wanted to 'smash someone or something'. He was discharged after 16 days and although he asked to see a psychiatrist, this was not arranged.

This example indicates that staff were apparently not attuned to the patient's emotional reactions to his illness and suggests that lack of support had led to grave distress. More time in conversation or just listening and more consideration may have alleviated this patient's feeling of isolation.

Case study no. 2

A 68-year-old woman was admitted for assessment of a cardiac condition with a view to surgery. She said she felt very anxious about coming into hospital and leaving her mentally retarded sister. However, it was imperative for her to get well so she gladly accepted the fact that she would be having tests and an operation. (Her GP had explained that she was admitted to this hospital in order to obtain the best cardiac surgery.)

After her cardiac catheter, Miss C was fairly content. This test was 'not so bad really'. The next few days were spent waiting for news of her test results and her operation. She missed her sister and cat and felt 'very lonely'.

She had several disturbed nights as the ward was very busy and she found it difficult to rest in the day-time because several patients were 'always laughing'.

During the second week Miss C complained that she did not know what was going to happen, when the operation was planned or if indeed she had been forgotten. On three occasions her doctors did a round but passed her by and she felt that they were neglecting her. She also felt rather sad that everyone around her seemed to be going home.

In the middle of this week a group of students arrived to listen to her chest but there was still no news. When she asked sister, she was told they were waiting for a vacancy on the operating list and on the intensive care unit. This did not really help her to be more optimistic.

On the fifteenth day the interviewer arrived to see Miss C's bed surrounded by three doctors. After they had left she was tearful and said she felt as upset and anxious and depressed as she could. They had told her that they considered it unwise to operate this time and that she should go home. So she unhappily made some plans.

The following day Miss C was not on the medical ward but had been transferred prior to her operation. Apparently a vacancy had been found on the list. Two weeks later Miss C was visited on the surgical ward after a 'very difficult' post-operative recovery.

Once more this vignette, giving the patient's side of the picture, shows how desperate someone can be when they are so dependent on staff for information. Through not keeping Miss C informed and not keeping in touch with her feelings staff were adding to the stress of major surgical treatment.

In attempting to prevent such instances, the final Chapter reviews ways for preventing unnecessary stress in hospital. Some, but not many, guidelines for giving psychological care are provided from research findings. These, too, are examined. Where this kind of evidence does not exist the author may resort to documented opinions which are widely held yet still have to be tested.

Signs of early emotional disturbance and maladaptive patient behaviour are also discussed, as nurses, in particular, can be invaluable in observing and evaluating their patients' responses. Recognition and awareness of the prevalence of early psychological morbidity with physical illness may promote earlier intervention and prevent severe psychological problems which hamper physical recovery. Research has exposed the enormity of the problem and the many deficiencies in care. It may now be most constructive to evaluate some of the suggestions which might alleviate distress and help patients cope with illness.

1

Stress as a precursor to illness

An artificial separation has developed between the psychological and physical processes in the practice of health care. This false dichotomy is reflected in the present-day use of the word 'stress' (originally an aphetic form of 'distress') as a psychological phenomenon and the word 'disease' (= dis-ease) as a physical one, since originally they had fairly closely related meanings. Recent work in psychobiology and a growing emphasis on and interest in psychosomatic medicine confirm how closely the two are related.

DEFINITIONS OF STRESS

Before discussing how the experience of stressful episodes seems to predispose to illness and how illness itself is related in turn to alteration of psychological processes some definitions are required.

It is important to understand initially that there is a close relationship between the concept of stress and so-called 'negative emotions', such as anxiety and depression. Some authors use the term psychological stress to refer to anxiety and depression. Others, while recognising both stress and anxiety are responses to threat, indicate that stress is experienced as a cognitive process rather than an emotional one (e.g., Lazarus, 1967).

Sociological studies of 'stress' frequently include descriptions and analyses of environmental events. Thus terminology tends to differ from that used by psychologists and psychiatrists who are more involved with the intra-personal rather than interpersonal experiences. This may explain why stress is often used as a fairly broad concept and lacks much integration with work on negative emotions.

Because 'stress' has been used by different disciplines it has come to have three meanings. Firstly stress can refer to an external threat which elicits a response of 'strain'. Used in this way it is a clear extension of physical principles (e.g., Langer and Michaels, 1963). The other two meanings, in contrast, describe the individual's response as stress. One definition sees stress as a reaction to threat.

For instance, Janis (1958) describes three phases of stress. Initially there is a threat phase where perception of danger arouses anticipatory fear. This is followed by the impact of the danger assessed in relation to escape and/or defenses which can be employed. The last phase is the post impact victimisation phase in which losses are perceived and deprivation is felt. This stage is associated with other emotions such as depression.

The second and quite similar use of stress as the reaction to an event is employed by Selye (1956). He also divided stress reactions into three stages; awareness, resistance when maximum adaptation occurs and lastly when stress persists, exhaustion and a state of physical and psychological disease. Since his early days of research in this area Selye has viewed stress situations as those which require adjustment by the organism. The situation may be pleasant or unpleasant, it is the intensity of the demand for adjustment behaviour that is the significant aspect of the situation.

Selye's contribution to knowledge, from a medical and experimental background, is important. His observations of animals and humans under stress were described as the general adaptation syndrome (GAS). From the alarm or awareness stage to exhaustion he recorded such signs as palpitations, tachycardia, tremors, weakness and insomnia and accounted for these in terms of sympathetic nervous system activation. During the resistance and adjustment stages this activation ceases and homeostasis is restored. If subjects cannot cope adequately, most likely when stress is prolonged, exhaustion and morbidity occur.

Recent ideas on stress integrate both adaptive responses and other responses, not necessarily adaptive, which relate specifically to threatening events. Ruff and Korchin (1967) view stress as the effort to maintain essential functions and the actual adjustment or adaptation required by the organism to tolerate any extra load. Stress, for them, involves modification of activities, adaptation and a compensatory response. Likewise Lazarus (1967) emphasised that stress reactions are reflections or consequences of the individual's appraisal of a situation and of his ability to act accordingly.

A more clinical approach to the subject is taken by Engel (1970) who describes three types of events which are usually considered as stressful. He discusses 'loss' or 'exit' events as stressful, particularly when they relate to an important person, role or ideal. The second major type of stress he mentions is injury to the body. Whether this is actual or only threatened it can cause great anxiety and other psychological morbidity. Thirdly, stress is related to repeated or continual frustration of drives, either for basic requirements like food or sex or more sophisticated ones such as career achievement.

Similar events and reactions to these were mentioned by Lipowski (1975). He suggested as being stressful the 'disorienting rate of social change; value, choice and decision conflicts, wants created by the existing economic system, coupled with aroused expectations and inability to meet them; status inconsistency. . .'.

THE RELATIONSHIP OF STRESS TO 'NEGATIVE EMOTIONS'

At each stage of a stress response a person may experience certain emotions. Awareness of a threat or an event requiring adjustment may evoke anxiety. This feeling may be related to thoughts of bodily harm or to feelings of inadequacy of ability to cope with the demands of the event. At a later stage anxiety about the effectiveness of adjustments made or about recurrence of the event may occur, or, alternatively, if the subject is unable to cope depression or grieving over the failure may result.

Terms used to describe feelings or emotions are particularly difficult to discuss but unless we have some knowledge of what is meant by 'anxiety' or 'depression' we cannot start to understand patients who experience these emotions and attempt to give help. Both anxiety and depression are collectively described as negative emotions, moods, or affective responses. They describe feelings or subjective experiences and as they are the major concepts used when describing emotional distress, they will be explained in more detail here.

Anxiety has been defined by Spielberger (1972) as 'a transitory emotional state or condition characterised by feelings of tension and apprehension and heightened autonomic nervous system activity'. Related to an event in the future, it is akin to fear, but it is said to be disproportionate to the 'threat' and is often in response to something which is 'unknown'. It is generally recognised to be a complex of other emotions such as fear, distress, guilt, surprise and fatigue (Izard, 1972).

The physical signs associated with subjective feelings of anxiety are closely related to general arousal caused by sympathetic nervous stimulation. Muscle tension, restlessness, incoordination and freezing may be felt initially, but if the emotion is prolonged, flushing, sweating, anorexia, hyperventilation, palpitations and diarrhoea may occur. In a chronic state of anxiety many changes in thinking occur, such as reduced concentration, distractibility, forgetfulness, irritability, insomnia and perceptual disturbance.

Descriptions of the subjective and physical feelings of anxiety are obviously very similar to the responses described in many stressful situations. Just as there is a variation in individuals' propensity to describe and respond to a stressful situation, there is also a variation in their proneness to feel anxious. Levitt (1971) points out that when describing a person as anxious it is essential to differentiate between whether a person is anxious as a temporary response to a situation or whether they are often anxious. In the latter case an anxious 'trait' will form part of the personality structure of that individual; in the former there is a 'state' of anxiety as a response to a situation or event.

This differentiation between state and trait also applies to descriptions of depression. Depression, like anxiety, is seen as a dysphoric mood or emotion, which may result after stressful episodes (Paykel, 1974). There tends to be withdrawal and lethargy accompanying feelings of worthlessness but also sometimes guilt and anxiety (Izard, 1972). It is therefore another complex of feelings which may persist for a long period and may be extremely severe or be experienced as a temporary feeling of 'the blues'. Physical concomitants are less easy to detect and explain but fatigue, anorexia, insomnia, constipation and weight loss may be present in a chronic state. That somatic accompaniments do occur, however, is well recognised and the term somatic depression or masked depression is used clinically to describe such phenomena (Kielholz, 1973).

THE RELATIONSHIP OF STRESS AND DISEASE MECHANISMS

Individuals' perceptions of what is stressful is very varied. Some people feel continually threatened by situations or events that do not affect others. In the same way, certain people become ill in the face of slight stress while others remain healthy under the same conditions. A predisposition to fall ill under stress may also be associated with a predispositon for certain types of illness. Explanations for the genesis of such an illness tend to be complex and usually include an interactive process between environmental and personality factors (often in conjunction with the presence of an external pathogen or irritant) such as the relationship represented in Figure 1.

Information on the interaction between stress reactions and physical changes associated with illness has been gained from research with both animals and humans. It has been possible to demonstrate with animals that the stress of a painful or fear-promoting situation produces physical changes. Much of this research has provided logical explanations for the mechanisms which produce disease and also how stress, seen as both an adaptive response and a response to threat with

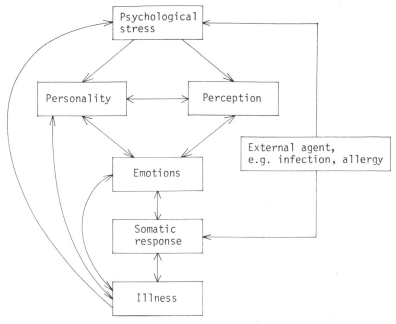

Fig. 1

lack of adaptation, has been associated with morbidity.

Selye did much of the pioneering work in this field. In the 1950s he administered high doses of corticosteroid hormones to animals and demonstrated resulting pathology of the heart and kidneys, which was extensive. He reasoned that repeated doses of these hormones would mimic the effect of constant stress and this showed that the physiological responses could lead to tissue damage.

Selye's further work was designed to show that low levels of 'stress hormones' are adaptive but abnormally high levels of these substances are associated with acceleration of disease. To show the effects of corticosteroids on the inflammatory and traumatic response of tissue to injury, he injected rats with an oil substance into a subcutaneous space. He compared the rapid healing processes in a group of normal rats with the lack of healing and increased trauma in rats who were given high doses of corticosteroids.

Other experiments have been undertaken to assess how environmental stresses affect health. Brady (1958) described an experiment on monkeys which were given repeated electric shocks while in restraining chairs. Those monkeys that were able to prevent the shock by pressing a lever (the 'executive' monkeys) were found to develop peptic ulcers, whereas those who were given a dummy lever did not develop them. Intermittent shock periods and rest periods were given and Brady found that rise in gastric acid secretions occurred in the rest periods. Without these rest periods the executive monkeys did not develop ulcers. They concluded that the ability to prevent shocks in a learned way was shown to be more stressful than being a recipient of these shocks. Conger, Lawrey and Turrell (1958), however, found that the efficacy with which an unanticipated series of electric shocks, in previously conditioned animals, can produce peptic ulcers is determined to a large extent by whether the animals are shocked in isolation (resulting in high ulcer rates) or in the presence of litter mates (resulting in low ulcer rates).

Liddell (1950) found that a kid isolated in an experimental chamber and subjected to a monotonous conditioning stimulus developed signs of 'experimental neurosis', consisting of cowering in the corner, trembling and an increased frequency of defaecation and micturition. While the twin, in an adjoining chamber, accompanied by its mother, exposed to the same stress, did not develop any of these signs. From this evidence on animals it seems that the effects of stress are considerably reduced when 'related' animals are present.

The particular effect on animals' behaviour in relation to each other resulting in stress situations has also been studied. For instance, overcrowding of animals in captivity eventually leads to increased infant and maternal mortality. In addition, this causes a disorganisation in animals' usual relationships and behaviour. Their actions no longer elicit anticipated responses and this frequently results in autonomic arousal and disturbed behaviour (Calhoun, 1962). Studies such as these indicate that various situations, which can be described as stressful, result in high levels of morbidity in animals.

THE STRESS OF LIFE EVENTS AND ILLNESS ONSET

In humans also a series of stressful events has been recognised as a precursory condition to illness.

The occurrence of social events or changes, both pleasant and unpleasant, has been studied in relation to many illnesses. Most of these studies see the adjustment to changes or 'life events' as a component of stress and attempt to assess the level of premorbid stress by enumerating events which have occurred prior to a certain illness. For example, Rahe (1968) devised a schedule of recent life experiences, such as marriage, a new job, having a child, etc. and found that minor illnesses, in particular, seemed to be associated with a greater incidence of life changes. He also interviewed a sample of males about recent illness and life experiences. Certain events, assumed to require considerable adjustment and change in life style, were often found to precede a bout of illness. Other workers have found that more life events occurred in the six months prior to psychosomatic illness than for a controlled group (Paykel, 1974). These results confirmed those of Brown and Birley (1968) who found that a relatively high incidence of life events were associated with the onset of schizophrenia. Certain events where the subject had experienced 'loss' of some kind were apparently more strongly associated with illness. Similar life events and illness relationships have been found for subarachnoid haemorrhage (Penrose, 1972), depressive illness (Paykel, 1974) and a variety of physical illnesses (Rahe, McKean, and Arthur, 1967).

These studies, therefore, seem to indicate that events which alter aspects of the social environment, especially those which require adjustment to loss, precede many illnesses. Such adjustment or adaptation, when viewed in terms of psychological stress (described above) may, therefore, be an influential factor in the generation of disease processes.

The effects of stress on physiological mechanisms are complex. Arousal of the sympathetic nervous system results in increased metabolism, blood clotting and raised intravascular volume as well as insensible fluid loss. In turn this produces raised blood pressure, increased pulse and respiration rate and an increased level of blood sugar. Symptoms include decreased urinary output, weakness, and cardiac arrhythmias (Stephensen, 1977). With any form of pre-existing pulmonary, cardiovascular or diabetic condition, serious illness may result if stress persists. Carruthers (1969) has explained how these processes can be related to coronary heart disease: high arousal is associated with catecholamine production and release. The effect of this is a break down of fatty deposits leading to higher blood levels of free fatty acids and increased coagulability of blood and a reduction in the break down of fibrin. Clots are, therefore, more easily formed in atheromatous vessels.

One study which gives support to the concept that stress is related to coronary heart disease looked at pre-morbid stress levels of patients with myocardial infarction (Thiel, Parker and Bruce, 1973). Fifty patients were studied to assess their life events, life style and habits and compared with a matched group of control subjects. Divorce was found more frequently among the patients, they more often felt lonely, had more disturbed relationships with colleagues, had worked more overtime, suffered more sleep disturbances and experienced more feelings of nervous stress and depression. Vetter, Cay, Phillip and Strange (1977) also found that myocardial infarction patients with higher anxiety or other stress responses during hospitalisation were more likely than others to suffer from cardiogenic shock and heart failure which led to a higher mortality rate.

Theories of a 'coronary personality' have been derived from such observations on coronary patients' life style and behaviour (see Olmsted and Kennedy, 1975). The Type A personality is said to be more likely to be associated with coronary heart disease due to the frequent experiences of stress. These people are less able to tolerate frustration, are more ambitious and have greater need of palliatives such as alcohol or nicotine and frequently express concern over the pressure of work. Type B, unlikely to suffer from this condition, seem more placid, patient and able to cope with the demands on their time and energies.

A model for the processes involved between the reactions to stress and the consequent disease process was discussed by Rees (1976). He suggested that people who suffer from various conditions become predisposed to react to stressful episodes in a way which will excacerbate their physical condition. This is summarised in Figure 2, which indicates the links between stress and consequent somatic and autonomic sequelae.

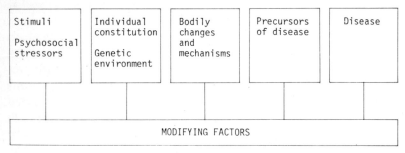

Fig. 2 The sequence of events from the psychosocial stressor to the disease process (from Rees, 1976, with permission).

In an extensive study of patients with disorders known to have a strong psychological component Rees found that there was a sizeable proportion who had suffered from a stressful episode prior to the onset of their illness (see Table 1). Bereavement and the grief reaction were found to be very powerful in terms of the distress and disability caused, as well as the physiological disturbances induced.

From this study he outlined the type of personality associated with psychogenic disorders. General instability, timidity, lack of self-assertion, anxiety proneness, marked sensitivity and obsessional attributes were included. But, he notes, 'the important fact is that all these traits of personality are in different ways conducive to development of states of emotional tension in response to environmental difficulties and these in turn may precipitate attacks of psychosomatic disorders'.

Table 1 Proportion of patients with pre-illness stress (from Rees, L. W. (1976) Stress, distress and disease. *British Journal of Psychiatry*, **128**, 3–18; with the permission of the Editor and author)

Disorder	%
Adult asthma	35
Vasomotor rhinitis	30
Hay fever	10
Urticaria	51
Thyrotoxicosis	44
Peptic ulcer	47.5

Stress reactions mediated by the sympathetic nervous system were shown by Selye (1973) to produce pathological reactions if continuous or extreme. Other chemical mediators such as histamine, acetylcholine, serotinin, catecholamines and prostaglandins may also be active in these processes and lead to cellular and organic change. Rees has explained that the effects of abnormally high levels of histamine and acetylcholine on local target organs, include contraction of smooth muscle, swelling of the mucosa, increased vascularity and capillary filtration and mucus secretion. All these are described in asthma, urticaria, hay fever, etc. and may be, therefore, the result of some increased secretion of one of the above.

Other evidence of psychosomatic links in stress comes from a recent study on bereaved subjects. It showed that there was an apparent alteration in the immune responses. Changes in the white cells had occurred which would render these people more vulnerable to infection. Such results suggest that the severe stress of recent bereavement may be associated with an increased propensity for illness (Bartrop, Lazarus, Luckhurst, Kiloh and Penny, 1977), and may explain the demonstrated increased morbidity and mortality in recently bereaved people (Parkes, Benjamin and Fitzgerald, 1969).

Much of previous animal work and the research on humans has been reviewed by Cassel (1974) who criticises the theoretical models of many stress studies. He sees the unitary relationship of a disease agent on the organism as over-simplified, for just as stressful situations may vary for each individual, so will the disease response. Stress, he suggests, is clearly not the only disease agent although it is contributory to most illnesses.

Cassel claims that one of the major stress contributors to illness is inadequate feedback or the lack of evidence that an individual's actions are leading to anticipated consequences. He points to vulnerable individuals who are of marginal status in society and thereby deprived of meaningful social contact, such as those who develop tuberculosis or schizophrenia, alcoholics, victims of multiple accidents and suicide. Immigrant groups are also highly likely to fall ill in unfamiliar surroundings, attempting to adjust but often deprived of the ability to communicate.

The effects of marginal status of new immigrants, exposed to high degrees of adjustment stress was the subject of Scotch's (1960) research. He measured blood pressure levels, as a physiological indicator of psychological stress among the Zulu who had recently migrated to urban centres and found they were significantly higher than in those Zulus in their original rural setting or those who had settled in the urban centres more than ten years previously.

Thus lack of meaningful interaction can be seen as stressful in itself but when this isolation is combined with further stress the effects on health are often severe. Further research with human beings has demonstrated this. For instance, Taylor, Wheeler and Altman (1968) subjected males to different conditions of isolation for several days. Isolated in pairs, they were either given separate cubicles for privacy but with a shared area or were placed together in a double-sized cubicle. Those in the first situation were not able to tolerate this for as long as the others and showed more stress reactions during the experiment. They concluded that total sharing and company was less stressful than a situation where there was opportunity for periods of isolation.

Nuckalls, Cassel and Kaplan (1972) studied how pregnancy affected women in relation to their system for social support. They assessed a sample of women in the thirty-second week of pregnancy with regard to accumulative life change and psychosocial assets or support. After delivery records were reviewed (blind) for any complications of pregnancy and delivery. 99 per cent of women with high life-change scores but low social assets had one or more complication, whereas only 33 per cent of women with equally high life-change scores but high social assets scores had any complications.

Similarly Brown's (1975) work on women living in an urban environment confirms that social support is an effective buffer against depressive illness. Those middle class women with children were able to establish a wider network of friends but were also more likely to have an understanding and supportive relationship with their husbands. In contrast, lower class women were much more likely to be 'trapped' at home with their children, unable to make friends and without much support or time spent with their spouse. This group had a significantly higher rate of depressive illness, related to a more stressful social situation and few support mechanisms to alleviate the harmful effects of this.

In conclusion, it appears there is substantial evidence that the experience of stressful episodes frequently precedes periods of illness. Stress may be an adjustment process or the reaction to some threat, both types may evoke anxiety. Certain individuals seem to experience more anxiety or stress than others. Stress, acting via established physiological mechanisms, leads to somatic change and morbidity. Some patients seem to have an illness proneness which is exacerbated by such stress. It seems that interaction with another is an important factor which alleviates the impact of stress and the absence of this interaction may in itself be stressful.

2

The onset of illness and reactions to it

It seems fairly widely accepted that patients react to illness with negative emotions. Literature, however, consists largely of documented opinions of physicians and psychiatrists, such as that of Lipowski (1975): 'Bodily injury or illness, or threat of either, constitute one of the major sources of psychological stress . . . illness itself includes psychosocial responses which may increase or reduce the initial psychological stress and thus influence the course and outcome of the illness'.

There are only a few systematic studies of patients' reactions and the situation has not greatly altered since Bartemeir (1961) said: 'Emotional reactions to illness may be described as the silent area in medical practice'. However, some of the factors influencing reactions are important when attempting to understand clinical situations and to help patients cope with illness.

Each individual's perception and acceptance of a symptom and of illness varies. The reasons for this are complex and, as yet, poorly understood. It may be said, however, that the final picture of an illness is the outcome of experience, personality characteristics and the different training the individual has had previously in respect of illness. These factors explain why it is that some individuals soldier on regardless and refuse to 'go sick', often further damaging their own health, while others seek help and report illness very readily, sometimes out of keeping with their symptoms. Some distinction may be drawn between illness – what the patient presents with – and disease – what the patient 'has'. Certain symptoms, for example, appear to have specific relevance. Mechanic (1962) found that vague complex symptoms, such as abdominal pain, were seen by the patient as more important than something which was localised and visible, like a sore finger, as the former could not be explained by the individual, who was then more likely to seek help. This initial desire to explain an illness was also stressed by Lipowski (1975). He recognised the nature or type of symptom or illness to be the fundamental influence for people to either take note of it or see it as nothing more than a nuisance. Thus bleeding, dyspnoea or pain could not be ignored whereas headaches, skin irritations and deafness could. Of course, there will also be individual variance regarding the severity of the symptom and when this is considered to need medical attention.

The importance attributed to a given symptom depends to some extent on the patient's knowledge of medicine and the body symptoms, on the person's resistance to carry on their normal behaviour with the symptom, and their life situation which may not allow them to even notice that something is amiss. Imboden (1972) discusses how some people deny the onset of an illness or symptom, especially if the onset is gradual. Deafness is a classic example of how people ignore signs that they are not hearing well and, accordingly, do nothing. Impairment of other sensory and cognitive abilities is also frequently ignored, as are psychiatric disturbances. Impairment of patients' thought or memory is frequently investigated only when others notice the change and initiate this (Imboden, 1972).

SEEKING MEDICAL AID

Knowledge of what disorder certain symptoms might indicate does not automatically result in rational action on the patient's part. Mechanic (1962) discusses what influences the decision to attend for medical consultation. The factors which influence a visit to the doctor are often not disease-related. For instance, his study with students showed that religion is influential in this. Protestants and Jews are far more likely to visit their doctor than Catholics or Christian Scientists. Why this should be so is unclear but he explained that studies have shown that, culturally, the former tend more to emphasise their pain experiences while the latter are more stoical. While these findings are based on American studies he suggests that an over-protective mother may act as a model for later health consciousness in her off-spring, a model which would be widely applicable. In addition, situational events were also found to affect medical consultations. Thus in a study of student attendance at a university health service, students who reported 'high' stress as measured by how frequently they were lonely and nervous, were more likely to use medical facilities. Mechanic found that during the time of study 60 per cent of high stress students visited the clinic three or more times as compared with only 38 per cent of the low stress students. As seen before, stress can be seen as a contributory factor to illness but it may also lead to a lowered tolerance of physical discomfort. Another factor which influences attendance for medical advice was found to be socio-economic status.

Early work in the United States showed that while upper-class people report themselves ill more often than those of the lower class, the latter actually suffer more symptoms (Koos, 1954).

Lipowski (1975) in an analysis of attitudes and expectations about illness and medical treatment, discussed the types of clinical disorder and symptomatology which were foremost in determining subsequent actions. Any symptoms which affect relationships are seen as important. Those which are visible or disfiguring are particularly likely to lead to medical consultation and when appearance is highly important to the individual even small disfigurement may result in quite severe psychological discomfort. Plastic surgeons are used to seeing such individuals who present with hardly noticeable blemishes which are affecting their social life and self-esteem adversely. In relation to this, secondary sexual organs when affected by a disorder are usually of great importance as a symbol of sexuality which might be threatened. Similarly, for someone with pride in their cleanliness, any degree of incontinence will, of course, be seen as a grave problem and medical aid will be sought rapidly. Thus, in anyone, their value system, personality and cultural background will determine when they accept a need for medical attention.

THE SICK ROLE

The original work on the sick role by Parsons (1951) clarified what was inferred by legitimisation of illness. He maintained that society had mechanisms for legitimising illness and to become sick in the eyes of others the patient must demonstrate his illness and it must be recognised by others as genuine and needing appropriate action. Subsequent to this recognition the sick person must respond to the need to get well.

Both Mechanic (1962) and Imboden (1972), adopting Parsons' ideas but adding a more medical dimension to his social model, referred to 'the sick role' as a type of appropriate behaviour which superseded other usual roles of mother, spouse, manager, etc. This new role implied exemption from responsibilities and an obligation to seek the help, comply with the advice of competent persons and then to surrender the sick role as soon as possible. As for sick-role behaviour, there are four options:

1. To adopt it and surrender it on recovery.
2. To reject or avoid it.
3. To adopt it readily and not give it up.
4. To strive to avoid it and then give in and cling to it.

These reactions to illness may depend on how much perceived pressure there is to sustain business and familial responsibilities. The wage-earner or the mother of a young child may be reluctant to accept or succumb to illness because of subsequent concern over their affairs, whereas someone else with worries and problems and possibly with fear of their inability to cope may readily relinquish their normal roles to become sick.

Normal reactions to illness
Thus adopting this 'sick role' is part of what is generally seen as acceptable behaviour. There are also other reactions to illness which are considered normal. On the whole, behaviour which is adaptive to a rapid recovery is considered normal, such as seeking timely medical advice, seeking for an explanation or reason for illness and compliance with therapeutic regimens and active information seeking about the treatment. Lipowski (1975) mentions the following as common reactions to illness, 'narrowing of interests, egocentricity, increased attention and responsiveness to bodily perceptions and functions, instability, an increased sense of insecurity and longing for human support and closeness'. Acute illness, he says, is usually accompanied by dependence, confinement and uncertainty.

The various difficulties patients have in dealing with the sick role is one of the determinants of their emotional responses to illness. Literature on this subject mainly involves hospitalised patients.

Emotional reactions to illness
Swift (1962) suggests that certain fundamental factors influence patients' reactions to illness. She includes the nature and severity of the illness, the age of the patient, the premorbid personality of the patient, previous experiences and the environmental circumstances and social system in which it occurs. These variables resemble those influencing the response to stress outlined above and Engel (1962) thus conceives of threat to the body or illness as a particularly severe form of psychological stress. Responses to this psychological stress may include the formation of an unpleasant affect, or sequence of affects, such as anxiety, guilt, hopelessness, helplessness, shame, disgust. Pathological, long-lasting, affective states associated with bodily changes also occur. The possible mechanism for this has been discussed above (p. 13).

However, much of this observation on reactions has been undertaken by psychiatrists in a consultant capacity among general hospital patients with grave psychological problems. Extreme reactions are, therefore, more likely to be emphasised. For example,

Lipowski (1967) says, 'From the nosological viewpoint, psychological reactions to organic disease spread over the whole spectrum of neuroses, psychoses and personality disorders'. Using a more general perspective he also admits (1975) 'The emotional responses to illness vary in quality, intensity and duration. They both reflect and influence the personal meaning of illness, the nature and degree of symptoms and disability, and the degree of support the patient gets from his environment. Anxiety, grief, depression, shame, guilt, anger – these are the affects most often elicited. Less common are apathy, indifference, elation or euphoria'. It is suggested that such reactions occur in many illnesses and situations. He traces stages of illness reactions which are commonly manifested:

1. The threat reaction to illness which is suspected or diagnosed in which anxiety and fear are dominant.
2. The symbolic loss accompanied by the realisation of illness and grief which may progress into a depressive syndrome. This may not be maladaptive; on the contrary, this may be necessary for acceptance and adjustment.
3. Gain may result after adjustment. A new meaning for the self endorsed by medical and others' attention may result in a new sense of self-importance.

Another psychiatrist, Schwab (1968), explains that anxiety will result as a reaction to illness if the patient has a premorbid disposition to anxiety states. In such a case the patient may become excessively anxious, any discomfort or pain being made worse by this reaction which may be unconsciously increased to exaggerate dependency needs. The anxious person also commonly reacts with hypochondriasis, somatisation, and even psychological invalidism. Similarly a naturally aggressive person may become a hostile patient resentful to unwanted dependency. Or, someone who is prone to repetitive or compulsive actions may become anxious or depressed in illness if they are unable to continue with their usual compulsive behaviour.

Byrne, Sternberg and Schwartz (1968) emphasise characteristic tendencies for people to act either as 'sensitisers' or 'repressors'. They suggest patients who are sensitisers will express reactions in one form or another, commonly mentioning discomfort and pain and complain of various aspects of care. Repressors, in contrast are likely to react to and perceive their illness differently. They commonly bottle up their feelings and tend to soldier on minimising their symptoms and emotions.

In general, there are a great variety of responses to illness and the simple dimension of repressor–sensitiser does not provide enough insight in the clinical setting. Schwab (1968) dealt with those reactions which are of particular concern to those in the caring professions. Some of these are discussed in brief below.

Regression

This term refers to a certain pattern of behaviour which is less adult or responsible than is usual for that person. Some degree of regression occurs for most patients who have to be looked after by others. Any limitation in activities usually means that, as with a child, preoccupation with self takes place. This, at first, is helpful for cooperation with the professionals but if it persists it complicates recovery and hampers resumption of previous adult roles.

Denial

Denial indicates a very fragile personality as it infers that acceptance of illness would threaten the integrity of the person and their ability to cope with everyday life. It can be very dangerous in some conditions. If early symptoms of a malignant disorder are 'denied', effective medical intervention is not possible. Titchener and Levine (1960) found that denial was sometimes responsible for delay in consenting to surgery for treatment of cancer until the condition was inoperable. Aitken-Swan and Paterson (1955) had also found this. They explained that if symptoms are perceived correctly or incorrectly as having ominous, life-threatening significance the patient may be so fearful he will tend to avoid examination. 45 per cent of their cancer patients were reported to have delayed for three months or more.

Refusal to accept illness or treatment often means difficult relationships with doctors. Patient and doctor disagree, the patient is uncooperative and this often leads him to take his own discharge against medical advice. When the 'denial reaction' is shattered Schwab says that psychosis or open hostility may appear.

Over-dependency

Over-dependency often results from a previous life of feeling isolated and rejected. This tends to prolong illness behaviour and leads to difficulties during rehabilitation. These patients tend to abuse their sick role by becoming too demanding. To some degree most sick people manipulate others for their own reward but this is only tolerated when others consider they are sufficiently sick to do so!

Although each individual reacts differently to illness a study attempting to generalise about patients' reactions in medical wards by Goldman and Schwab (1965) was fairly productive. They recognised four general types of patients:

1. The very ill, often terminally ill patients who frequently had highly rigid and unrealistic attitudes of denial. This was supposedly to prevent the necessity of considering the consequences of illness.
2. The moderately ill patients who assessed their illness as a nuisance – not involving the core of their lives. The temporary handicap was considered realistically which enabled them to cope.
3. Those with vague reactions who often complained about their illness but denied anxiety. They were often ambivalent, contradictory and less specific about their illness than other patients.
4. Those who were psychiatrically ill and were highly anxious and desperate to get well. Often they expressed wishes to radically change their life pattern if deemed therapeutic.

To avoid the need to categorise in this way Pilowsky (1975) has contained all varieties of abnormal behaviour related to illness as 'abnormal illness behaviour'. He explains that premorbid personality, cultural and social factors determine the 'illness behaviour', emotional and behavioural responses to illness to a greater extent than the illness itself. Abnormal illness behaviour needs, therefore, to be recognised and treated in terms of the variety of a particular patient's needs for adjusting to illness.

There is evidence of a high rate of psychological morbidity in general ward patients. Psychiatrists who receive requests for patient consultations have expressed the view that it is those patients who present as major treatment problems or with distressing or aggressive behaviour who are usually referred. In other words, when staff experience difficulty in coping with these patients they ask for assistance. Patients who do not manifest their reactions in this way are less likely to receive help, although they may need it. Quiet, extremely anxious and depressed patients are frequent examples in this group.

Moffic and Paykel (1975) studied 150 general-ward in-patients and found 24 per cent with an above normal degree of depression. The incidence of depression was commoner in those with more severe medical illness, more concomitant stress and more previous depression. Schwab, Bidlow, Brown and Holzer (1967) described the behaviour and feelings of their depressed general ward in-patients. They found that the type of depression was qualitatively different to that found in a psychiatric population and indicated that its presentation picture was related to social class. Apathy or active seeking for help and clinging to the 'real' world were characteristic for these general patients. However, socio-economic class 5 patients tended to present as 'a futility syndrome' with passivity and 'a given up' attitude.

EMOTIONAL REACTIONS IN RELATION TO PHYSICAL DISORDERS

Certain illnesses are considered to be more likely to produce emotional reactions and complications than others. The reasons for this are not clear. Lipowski (1967) reviews evidence showing that viral infections such as hepatitis, are usually followed by depression. Castelnuovo-Tedescu (1961) listed many other disorders complicated by depression, including cardiac conditions, ulcerative colitis, asthma, neurodermatitis, anaemia, malignancies and endocrine disorders. Central nervous system diseases in particular, such as epilepsy or multiple sclerosis, also appear to be positively associated with emotional disorders (Merskey and Trimble, 1979).

Chronic illness has been found to result in varying emotional reactions. Brown (1950) found indifference and apathy as the main symptoms in chronic illness. Whereas Starrett (1961) found long term paraplegic patients displayed permanent defenses such as denial, hostility and depression, although the initial onset of the condition was associated with high levels of anxiety caused by disruption of the body image.

In the case of patients with kidney failure other organic factors also alter mood states, such as salt depletion. Neary (1976) reviews recent data which suggests that depression was the commonest reaction to renal failure. Anxiety and irritability occurs in at least a third of chronic ureamics. Neary also mentions methyldopa (a hypotensive agent) as precipitating depression for this group of patients. Drugs seem a potent source of emotional disturbance in association with illness. Lloyd (1977) mentions reserpine, levodopa, atropine and anti-tuberculous drugs, in particular, although the list of drugs with psychological side effects grows daily.

In these cases anxiety and depression may be a predominant sign of a physical illness. The alternative relationship between depression and physical symptoms, namely physical symptoms as a manifestation of depression, has been the subject of a conference, the proceedings of which were edited by Kielholz (1973). Contributors noted the prevalence of somatisation of depressive illness and the frequent presentation of physical symptoms which were helped by anti-depressant therapy. These ideas serve to highlight the dynamic interaction between physical and psychological functions and suggests how both may be impaired by stress.

THE EFFECT OF ILLNESS ON THE FAMILY

Dynamics of normal inter-personal relationships are obviously changed when a family member contracts an illness. Whether the patient is nursed at home or is withdrawn from the family to be cared for in hospital, change in the roles of the remaining members will probably occur.

Lipowski (1975) observed that long term illness, in particular, led to family discord, often related to increased problems financially. Despite social security (in this country) self-employed earners have suffered financially by even short term illnesses, and long term plans for expenditure also had to be altered if a wage earner was ill (French, Sutherland, Mitchell and Mossman, 1977). If the 'bread winner' is sick the wife often has to work as well as care for her husband, this extra strain readily leads to a decline in marital concord. Any disharmony in the marriage may well be accentuated, as may be the wife's own dependence/independence conflicts.

Little research has been done on the family's response to illness in one of the members. However, Freidman, Chodoff and Mason (1963) undertook some insightful work with the parents of leukaemic children. They monitored their stress reactions on physiological and psychological parameters. Parents' reactions were traced through the following:

1. Shock and an inability to comprehend.
2. A tendency to self-blame with guilt feelings for imaginary errors in omission and neglect at the onset of symptoms.
3. An information-seeking period in an attempt to control the disease.
4. Hope for cures and remission.
5. Anticipatory grief.

Many of these reactions, of course, mirror those of patients when reacting to illness themselves.

CONCLUSION

It is suggested that emotional responses to illness are varied and present intermittently. In that most studies are hospital-based and concentrate on more serious illness the more extreme emotional and behavioural reactions have been discussed here. However, health workers, and perhaps nurses, have most opportunity to detect early signs of maladaptive responses to illness. Without knowledge of some of the problems and precipitating factors early signs of distress and even pathology may be missed, thus preventing any intervention and corrective action. Emotional reactions in themselves should sometimes be seen as inevitable in the face of illness but when they prevent rehabilitation they obviously become a grave complication.

3

Admission and adjustment to hospital

Many people have maintained that admission to hospital is a key event which is usually accompanied by emotional reactions on the part of patients. Rachman and Philips (1975) listed five commonly-encountered manifestations of this stressful event, namely anxiety or fear, increased irritability, loss of interest in the outside world, unhappiness and preoccupation with one's bodily processes. While these may, of course, be seen as reactions to illness as well as hospitalisation, the events which occur during the admission process are thought to add to the distress and thus deserve discussion in their own right.

If one pictures the events which often precede admission to hospital, it is not surprising that negative emotional reactions, such as anxiety, occur. A period of illness or suspected disease must reduce the individual's resistance to further life stress, as coping with the onset of illness can be seen as a major adjustment. This fatigue and lowered coping ability is then not the ideal condition for facing the added stress of hospitalisation.

'Not knowing what to expect', 'anticipating the worst yet hoping it will not happen', 'wanting to fit in and feel comfortable yet not knowing what to do' must all combine to lead to anxious feelings. Robinson (1972) suggests that a patient will react to hospitalisation in the way he usually reacts or copes with any other stressful event and his usual defence mechanisms against anxiety feelings will be employed. Thus, if he usually trusts people the hospital staff will be trusted but they will also arouse his anger or hostility and be criticised if this is his usual approach.

Robinson describes the procedures of admission which she says give cues to patients about the priorities of the staff. These usually give cause for concern rather than reassurance for the patient. The name-band, for instance, which is used in many hospitals encourages staff to check the patient's name at a glance rather than by enquiry. This leads the patient to conclude that his intellectual processes are of lessened importance. The gown which emergency patients are given is usually standard or institutional so that the individual becomes another patient like so many others. The fact that patients routinely admitted are usually asked to get into bed immediately on admission may also give them the initial impression that 'the hospital' prefers them to fulfill their role as patient as soon as possible.

The fact that so many procedures have to be accepted by the individual on admission also points to the lack of individual initiative and rights for the patient. Robinson explains how the prodding and poking of medical examination, the collection of specimens and of personal information would not be tolerated outside hospital. Yet staff expect patients to submit to such things in a very matter-of-fact way. Their total orientation to the bodily processes may well give the impression that the patient's thoughts and feelings are of no importance to them. Goffman (1961) showed that in psychiatric hospitals the situation was very depersonalising. He suggested the rituals involved in admission rapidly turned the individual into another inmate who looked the same as others. Tolerance of this situation only came from internalising this role and 'becoming the same'. Although in a modern general hospital this description may seem extreme, it is useful to remember that for a patient in a heightened state of arousal each event will be interpreted very sensitively and perhaps abnormally. Patients learn that their bodily symptoms are of most importance and their needs are most effectively met if they can be channelled or communicated as physical complaints.

Levitt (1975) interviewed 200 general-ward patients in a large teaching hospital on how they responded to admission to hospital. The majority of patients usually accepted and were grateful for the care and attention given to them. She interpreted this as an adaptive passivity necessary to prevent a perpetual feeling of anxiety. This reaction to admission led to a great reluctance to ask staff questions as 'they were so busy' and thereby a reduced opportunity to adjust to hospitalisation and benefit from some of the facilities.

Children have been described as particularly emotionally vulnerable on admission. The classical studies of Spitz (1946) indicated how profoundly depressed and withdrawn children became during periods of hospitalisation. The lack of affection and social stimulation from staff was thought to cause long-standing psychological illness in these children. The relationship between reduced interaction and consequent depression is now widely accepted. In reviewing the work in this field, Rachman and Philips (1975) show that despite government committee reports that children's distress decreases if they are admitted accompanied by their mother, many hospitals do not provide facilities and still seem to discourage open visiting. Stacey's (1970) study showed that nurses considered their most important functions were to wash, dress and feed the children, not to play with or talk to them. If the major cause of upset for children is the unfamiliarity with the surroundings it would seem imperative that normal and pleasurable activities should be maintained, especially if the parents are not available. The vulnerable children were those who were uncommunicative, isolated, shy, very young or children without brothers or sisters. Stacey also found that anxiety from the parents on admission was transferred to children, so reassurance and attention to both the parents and child was necessary to reduce the stress of admission.

STUDIES OF ANXIETY OF NEWLY ADMITTED PATIENTS

Relatively few systematic studies of emotional responses to admission have been completed. A major problem of such studies is that reports of patients' views and feelings always depend on willingness of respondents to express their feelings. However, at present there is no other satisfactory way of obtaining this information.

An early interview study by Hugh Jones, Tanser and Whitby (1964) with 275 patients admitted to one medical firm in a London teaching hospital attempted to assess patients' views. This was a three-stage study, patients being interviewed twice while in hospital and once after their discharge from hospital. The interviewers were staff of the hospital and the authors did not claim this to be a representative study. They found that 46 per cent of their waiting-list patients were either 'anxious' or 'anxious and relieved' on admission, while only 34 per cent of the emergency admissions responded in this way. However, this may be a biased sample as a much larger proportion of emergency patients were unable to be interviewed at this initial stage. The type of worries the patients reported were very mixed but ranged from specific fears of hospital treatment to worries about their jobs. Men were more worried about outside concerns than the women patients.

REDUCTION OF ANXIETY

An American team of nurses, Elms and Leonard (1966) tested and upheld a hypothesis that explanation about hospital routines, facilities, procedures and information about patients' own illness and treatment reduced anxiety feelings on admission. This obviously relates to the idea that anxiety, seen as fear of the unknown, is reduced when more knowledge is given to the patient. Moran (1963) undertook a similar study with children awaiting tonsillectomy. She gave a full explanation of hospital procedures to children and their parents. Those patients who were prepared in this way were found to accept and adjust to hospital more easily than others. A similar hypothesis was proposed by Franklin (1974) in her work, *Patient Anxiety on Admission to Hospital*. This study will now be discussed in more detail as the aims were very relevant to this topic and to the dynamics of nursing care.

Franklin attempted to measure anxiety and the quality of nursing care and determine whether there was a relationship between these variables. The sample of 160 patients was drawn from surgical wards of four London hospitals. Quality of care was only assessed by patients' opinions on this subject and how much information they were given on admission. Anxiety was measured by Cattell's (Institute of Personality and Ability Testing) trait test of anxiety. To vary the independent variable (the quality of care) staff on one of the surgical wards were informed of the full purpose of the study.

The results of this study must be viewed in the light of qualifications in the methods used. The independent and dependent variables were subject to contamination, in that those who are anxious and depressed tend to be more critical and see their world with more pessimism. Patients' comments about the nursing care would, therefore, be more likely to be critical if they were anxious. The measure of anxiety was also not appropriate as this assessed predispositions rather than temporary experiences of the emotion.

Responses to some of the interview questions are useful. Thirty-one patients were 'very worried', 59 were 'a little worried' and 70 were 'not worried' on admission. Reasons for worry were as listed in Table 2.

Table 2 Causes of patients' anxiety on admission to hospital

Cause of anxiety	%
Did not know what to expect	32
Worried about operation	31
Worried about anaesthesia	18
Worried about family	11
General dislike of hospitals	8

Although Table 2 suggests that patients have fairly well defined areas of concern, the interpretation may not be so clear as these were responses to the question 'what have you been mainly worried about?'. This question inferred that people usually have one major worry and the first three response categories cannot really be seen as discrete or separate.

ADMISSION TO PARTICULAR CLINICAL AREAS

Vetter, Cay, Philip and Strange (1977) studied a sample of 338 patients with coronary thrombosis or ischaemia admitted to either a coronary care unit or a general ward. They found that admission to a coronary unit did not cause more anxiety than admission to a general ward did. Women were more anxious than men and those who had not suffered from myocardial infarction were more distressed than those who had. One explanation for this may be due to the continuous pain during ischaemia which is not experienced after infarction. Additionally or alternatively the patient with ischaemia may receive less attention than known cases of infarction. It was interesting that in this study reports of high anxiety levels were associated with mortality. This may be accounted for by Carruthers' explanation, mentioned in Chapter 1, where raised levels of catechol amines are said to produce an increase in cardiac arrhythmias, myocardial irritability and an increased propensity to thrombosis.

In an attempt to explain further the factors of hospitalisation which produced negative emotional responses in patients, Wilson-Barnett and Carrigy (1978) monitored the daily emotional reactions of general medical ward patients from the time of admission until discharge. Using a mood adjective check list developed by Lishman (1972) and a short interview schedule to collect patients' views on events which they experienced, 202 patients in two large hospitals were sampled over a period of nine months. Each patient also completed the Eysenck Personality Inventory (EPI) (1964) as a trait test of emotionality. One objective was to see when adjustment to being in hospital defined by the absence of negative emotional reactions occurred. Anxiety and depression scores were obtained from patients within 24 hours of their admission and were found to be significantly higher than their average scores throughout their stay in hospital. This rise in scores occurred in a great majority of patients regardless of their emotionality trait category of high, medium or low. No overall difference in scores was found between those patients admitted as an emergency when compared to those from the waiting list. Sex and age categories, when compared for anxiety levels on admission also revealed no statistically significant differences. On open questioning 43 per cent of the patients reacted in a negative way to being admitted. Several reasons were usually given by each patient, such as not wanting to leave their family and a fear of hospitals and concern about their condition. When responses were analysed according to whether patients felt 'quite' or 'extremely' ill or only 'slightly' or 'not at all' ill, it was found those who did not feel so ill were more likely to feel more negative about their admission to hospital.

Some of these results are at variance with those of other studies. For instance there were no differences between anxiety levels on admission for emergency patients and those from the waiting list, whereas Hugh Jones *et al.* (1964) found that the waiting-list patients were more anxious. However, although not statistically significant, females were apparently more anxious on admission, and this did correspond with findings of Vetter *et al.* (1977).

ADJUSTMENT TO HOSPITAL

Adjustment, or loss of initial emotional reactions has also been studied. In the study described above by Wilson-Barnett and Carrigy (1978) patients' daily reports of their emotions were recorded and this enabled a longitudinal description of adjustment. What was demonstrated was an important relationship between the personality disposition (emotionality trait) and adjustment time. Those with high trait scores of emotionality took longer to adjust. Often it was five days or more before their level of anxiety fell to zero. This result suggests that those who have a highly emotional disposition will probably respond to admission with negative emotions which then persist for some time at the beginning of their stay. Others will initially report feelings of anxiety and unhappiness but will lose these feelings after a day or two.

Another study of adjustment to hospital was carried out by De Wolfe, Barrell and Cummings (1966). They examined male patients admitted for long term (over six weeks) treatment to a sanitorium. They attempted to elicit personality factors and individual factors influencing emotional adjustment to long term medical wards. 517 patients were included and given two sets of questionnaires. They found that on admission younger patients were more depressed and worried about their admission, as were the better educated and more intelligent patients. Those who were younger, had a more critical attitude to responsibility and a higher anxiety trait than others and were more likely to have a longer and more difficult adjustment to hospital.

A less structured approach (observation) to the study of adjustment in general wards was used by Coser (1965). She also gave valuable insight into inter-patient dynamics, describing how patients gradually adopt the norm and join the other patients in a sub-culture where humour plays a large part and which does not accept expressions of distress or dissatisfaction. If a patient cries or complains the other patients assume that they are self-important, whereas if misfortune becomes the subject of a joke it can be shared and adds to their feelings of security and equality. These reactions, it seems, are encouraged by nursing and medical staff.

The results of failing to adopt the usual pattern of patient behaviour which, as shown, may be dependent on a variety of factors, including personality factors, are shown by the study of Stockwell (1972) who observed and interviewed patients in general wards. Those who complained or who openly manifested signs of distress were punished by being ignored by staff. These 'unpopular patients', that is, those who were talked to least frequently, and were said to be the least favoured by nurses, tended to be older and to have been in hospital for a longer time than others. Reflecting perhaps their anxiety traits, this group also included those who had a psychiatric history or were 'overtly' unhappy. The effects that such loss of interpersonal contact could have on care cannot be underestimated. It could lead to further distress and psychological morbidity which in turn might complicate physical recovery. This then leads to a vicious circle. Thus, as Levitt (1974) says: 'For his own part the patient will make life more tolerable for himself in hospital by confining his conscious anxiety to the illness itself. He will accept all the controls and demands that the environment exerts on him, and he will cooperate willingly with whatever routines and procedures are in operation, in order to reduce his awareness of conflict or ambiguity . . . it is those patients who are less able to do this who are unable to make the transition from person to patient who consciously suffer more anxiety.'

The passive acceptance of hospitalisation is, therefore, part of adjustment to life as a patient. Asking questions and giving suggestions is seen by many patients, and some staff, as a nuisance to staff. Patients, therefore, tend to wait to be given information or pick it up from other patients. As such, their apprehension increases and their belief in myths about their illness is reinforced.

CONCLUSION

Findings from the research on patients' reactions to admission to hospital indicate that this is a very stressful event. Factors which generate anxiety include concern over the illness, what it might be and what treatment will be required. In addition learned fears of hospitals and concerns over what the doctors, nurses and patients will be like and a lack of knowledge about the new environment and role of patient create a complex of worries leading to insecurity and distress. Although this has been well documented, certain procedures which add to the stress, such as non-response from staff or the repetitious requests for information from patients and the removal of patients' clothes, continue. The ideal situation should be apparent. The hospital becomes the patient's home and as such should be a place of rest and harmony, not stress and frustration. Nurses, in particular, have a most important role at the time of a patient's admission. Their welcome to patients should be friendly, very polite and they should act fundamentally as an information source. In reality, it seems that the institutional needs are satisfied rather than those of the patient. This is very unfortunate as the newly-admitted patient's initial experience may well determine how he views his stay and his progress while in hospital.

4

Events in hospital and patients' reactions

Over the last two decades, research on how patients view their experiences in hospital has revealed very similar findings. The same aspects are mentioned as distressing or disliked throughout. This may be because there are inevitable consequences of admission to hospital or it may be that staff in the hospitals are either unaware of these problems or have not found remedies for the many things that make patients annoyed or unhappy.

FINDINGS FROM SURVEYS ON PATIENTS' OPINIONS

Early surveys by McGhee (1961) and Cartwright (1964) in Scotland and England respectively exposed many common areas of hospital life to which patients objected. Patients' dislikes included having to use bedpans, noise, especially of nurses' feet, doors banging and of other patients coughing, etc., the rigid routine, so many new faces, having to choose the right grade of nurse for the right request, being put into single rooms and having doctors talking over them using technical terms.

Patients also complained of unsatisfactory seating arrangements and seemed to benefit from a day room, perhaps to escape from the ward. They found that having their tea at visiting time was embarrassing and visiting hours were unnecessarily restricted. At night time everything seemed more dramatic and anxiety was reinforced by subdued lighting and whispering. Noises were, therefore, interpreted as boding strange happenings with sinister connotations. At the end of their stay many patients were discharged without much warning when their bed was required for another admission. This led to confusion for both patients and staff.

McGhee discussed, in particular, how lack of space and privacy distressed patients. They felt unable to hold a confidential conversation, as it would be overheard. This made them reluctant to discuss their fears or intimate worries. On the other hand when patients could discuss and communicate their needs this was seen to be positively therapeutic. Cartwright's (1964) research confirmed that psychological needs were neglected: 'While nurses look after patients' physical needs, and can encourage confidence or allay anxieties, they are often too busy or preoccupied to spend a great deal of time talking to patients. It is on their fellow patients that most people rely for companionship'.

When examining how anxieties could be alleviated Cartwright noted that patients could not obtain information easily from staff and that 44 per cent of patients said they obtained 'no' information from the Sister, 40 per cent 'a little', and only 16 per cent said they obtained 'a lot'. She suggested that middle class patients were more able to communicate with staff and therefore satisfy their needs, but this did not mean that working class patients needed less support or information, they were perhaps just less expressive of these needs.

Lack of information is a fairly common complaint in most surveys. Barnes (1961) reported the proceedings of an international conference and the views expressed at the congress included the distress felt by 'fear of the unknown' and the helplessness felt by being unable to glean information from staff who seemed busy and impersonal.

Hugh Jones, Tanser and Whitby (1964) sampled medical ward patients admitted under the care of two Consultants in a London teaching hospital. From this research they found that 41 per cent of men and 34 per cent of women were worried about being in hospital. Finance (39 per cent), business (25 per cent) and family responsibilities (25 per cent) were the most important worries. 21 per cent of these patients complained about noise. 20 per cent of the female patients who had been 'taught on' during a students' round disliked this, although only 5 per cent of the males objected to it. 27 per cent of the patients did not know who had visited them in a white coat. However, despite doctors' efforts to explain diagnoses, 39 per cent of patients were still dissatisfied with the amount of information, 65 per cent wanted more information and 3 per cent wanted less. There are many possible explanations for this dissatisfaction. It may have been patients' anxieties in the doctors presence which prevented them from understanding what he was saying or it may have been the doctor's incapacity to give clear information to these patients.

Results from Raphael's (1969) survey of over 1300 general-ward patients on their experience of hospital provided information on particular hospital facilities. The great majority of patients were generally more contented than discontented about their stay. However, younger patients tended to be more critical than others and females were also more critical than males. The items which patients most disliked were the sanitary facilities, the boredom, the noise at night and sleepless nights and the suffering and complaints patients.

A comparable study in the United States by Volicer and Bohannon (1973) had similar findings. Patients were asked to rank items on a list according to the amount of anxiety they caused. Financial worries were ranked high (which may have been a function of the American health insurance scheme); so also was inadequate explanation of treatment and diagnosis as well as the unconcerned attitude of the hospital staff. Changes in eating, sleeping and being away from work were rated very low on this scale. However, many extreme examples were also included, such as loss of a limb or disfigurement, which may alter patients' perspective in rating the more routine aspects of hospital life.

Another study by Wriglesworth and Williams (1975) studied the relationships between the various aspects of being in hospital to see if clusters of 'dislike' existed. Although their sample of 80 male surgical patients cannot be viewed as representative of general patients *per se*, some of the correlations appear meaningful. For instance, opinions about food correlated with aspects of comfort. Opinions of staff helpfulness, awareness and friendliness were related to what patients thought about the general atmosphere of the ward and also their degree of confidence in the staff. They said 'It appeared that the amount of information given to the patient and his resulting degree of confidence in the staff are inextricably bound up'.

A recent and on-going study in Scotland on patients' fears and worries by French, Sutherland, Mitchell and Mossman (1977) is examining fears and dislikes of general medical and surgical ward patients. The team interviewed patients within 48 hours of their admission and then after four or five days spent in hospital. Some of the main findings include patients' worries at seeing those who are more ill than themselves, having to have things done for them, their loss of freedom and difficulty in passing the time away (which was usually only expressed by patients at their second interview), and their general lack of adequate information about their condition and of tests and operation results.

In order to see which hospital events were most commonly liked and disliked an interview study was undertaken with medical-ward patients (Wilson-Barnett, 1976). Open questions on sixty aspects of hospital life were asked of 200 patients from two hospitals. These items were then ranked according to the number of patients who responded negatively or positively. Tables 3 and 4 give the ranked order of these items:

Significantly more negative than positive responses were given to

Table 3 Items which elicited predominantly negative responses from patients (n = 200)

Items	Positive	Neutral	Negative	Not applicable
Using a bedpan	3	29	130	38
Anticipating a treatment, or procedure which is likely to be painful	0	91	109	0
Seeing another patient who is very ill	2	89	106	3
Leaving your usual 'work' while you are in hospital	8	100	91	1
Being away from the family	10	97	85	8
Your own condition or illness	0	123	77	0

all these items in Table 3, as shown by the one sample chi-square test (1 d.f. at 1 per cent level).

Significantly more positive than negative replies were given to all the items in Table 4 as shown by the one sample chi-square test (1 d.f. at 1 per cent level).

The same items were found to be mentioned 'negatively' or 'positively' by most people in both hospital samples, lending a degree of generality to the results.

Six items stood out as regularly evoking negative responses (see Table 3). In addition to these, 'the night time' elicited 'negative' reactions from 86 people. They often felt it was difficult to sleep in a ward with the noises of other patients or they just felt 'strange'. Also 90 per cent of the patients who had experienced barium X-rays described the experience in negative terms, such as, apprehension, discomfort or embarrassment.

Far more items elicited positive responses than negative responses (see Table 4). Patients, on the whole, were grateful for and welcomed the attention they received in hospital.

As found with studies mentioned above there was a difference in responses from sub-groups in this sample. Thus, there was an overall tendency for females to give more negative responses than males and for the younger patients (i.e., those under 40 years) to give more negative responses than those of 40 and over. Four exceptions to this trend were found. For instance, older patients gave more negative responses to 'having television on in the ward', and all males expressed more negative replies to 'being away from your family'. When the attitudes of all older patients to 'your own discharge from

Table 4 Items which elicited predominantly positive responses from patients (n = 200)

Items	Positive	Neutral	Negative	Not applicable
Early-morning tea	160	18	18	4
Talking to the staff nurse	148	45	6	1
Your own discharge from hospital	146	31	23	0
Teatime	141	41	16	2
Talking to the student nurses	140	48	2	10
Lunchtime	135	31	33	1
Being able to have the odd nap	135	46	15	4
Talking to your visitors	134	38	11	17
Supper	130	35	32	3
Sister's round, when she comes on duty	129	55	7	9
Talking to your consultant	122	51	7	20
Talking to your (junior) doctor	121	55	23	1
Breakfast time	116	39	42	3
Having set visiting times	112	53	31	4
Being able to have a private conversation with your relatives when they visit	111	54	19	16
Talking to other patients	102	65	32	1
Your admission to this ward	96	63	38	3
The work of the night nurses	95	85	13	7
The smoking restrictions	95	74	31	0

hospital' were compared, it was found that more females replied negatively. One other finding concerned attitudes to 'the doctor's round' – when the under 40s' replies were compared between the sexes, males gave more negative responses.

The main findings of this study were unequivocal and support the findings from other studies. Patients gave many more positive than negative responses to inquiry about their reactions to a long list of items relating to their stay in hospital. This implies that patients had generally positive feelings and attitudes towards ward events. It would, however, be surprising if social desirability and other misleading response sets did not prevent most people giving at least a few negative responses. The finding that females gave more negative responses than males could be explained in many ways. It could be considered more socially acceptable for females to express emotions such as fear or unhappiness than males who are socialised not to express such emotions. It could, however, be a reflection of more psychiatric disability and depression among women or the possibility that the female medical wards have a more depressing or distressing atmosphere. Also the activities in the ward are somewhat 'domestic', such as cleaning, bedmaking and meal-serving. As this is traditionally the female realm of interest one might expect them to have critical ideas on the subject.

The fact that younger patients gave more negative replies confirms many of the previous studies' results. It suggests that their attitude of increased concern and criticism denotes a more assertive role as patient.

In relation to information discussed above, one quarter of the patients surveyed mentioned feelings of unease about not having information concerning their progress or with regard to their role and what was expected of them in certain situations. With regard to diagnostic tests they mentioned feelings of 'fear of the unknown'.

A problem with interpretation of these results is the individual 'personality' or consistent attitude to some of the questions which seemed to be a dominant factor influencing responses. Some individuals gave several negative replies (between 30 or 40) while the majority gave very few (under 10). As mentioned before, personality factors influence reactions to illness, the sick role and recovery, and it seems important, therefore, to assess how patients' personality factors influence their reactions to events in hospital.

An attempt to assess how personal, medical and personality factors effect reactions to certain events in hospital has been undertaken and will be discussed more fully (Wilson-Barnett and Carrigy, 1978). The aims of the study were as follows:

1. To explain when emotional reactions occur during a patient's stay in hospital and what aspects of hospital life influence these.
2. To examine which types of patients react to which sort of hospital life.
3. To pin-point those patients most likely to experience most feelings of anxiety and depression.

Data were collected from two hospitals. Over thirteen hundred interviews were carried out with 202 patients. As explained in the previous Chapter, they were interviewed daily using two instruments, one to record mood, the other their responses to events in hospital. The first was a mood adjective check list (Lishman, 1972) and the second was a list of items which were previously shown to elicit most 'negative' reactions (Wilson-Barnett, 1976). Patients were asked how they had felt for the last 24 hours and to complete the adjective check list accordingly. Then, using the item list as focus for a brief interview, patients were asked whether the items had affected them and in what way. They were also asked to give an indication of how unwell or well they had felt on a four-point rating scale. In addition, each patient completed an EPI (Eysenck and Eysenck, 1964), so that emotionality and extroversion traits could be related to other findings.

Patients' responses in regard to their illness or condition were recorded and assessed in two ways. Firstly emotionality scores were correlated with illness ratings. There was no overall statistical relationship between the degree of physical illness and feelings of emotional distress. Secondly, the patients were grouped according to a diagnostic classification and it was found that patients in the psychosomatic, infective and neoplastic categories had higher average anxiety and depression scores (see Table 5), although there were only small numbers in some categories and the results were not statistically significant.

In addition to these emotionality ratings, patients were asked how they felt about their condition and progress and the proportion of negative comments was calculated. Certain patients were found to be more concerned about their condition, and those in the neoplastic or infective groups gave more negative replies than others but the 'undiagnosed' or 'other category' patients also expressed concern. This was usually attributed to fears of what was causing their illness, to wondering if the doctors thought they were hypochondriacs and to not being able to justify to others reasons for their hospitalisation.

The longitudinal design of this study enabled a trend of comments to be outlined. For instance 29.9 per cent of patients expressed concern about their condition at the beginning of their stay but after treatment or consultation felt much less concerned. As can be seen from Table 5, just over a third of all the comments were in some way negative. In fact 86.1 per cent of all patients made at least one such comment. Those who made most of these comments of concern were of a higher emotional disposition or were in the younger age range, that is, under 40 years of age.

From this study several other aspects emerged which were found particularly distressing for certain patients. These will now be discussed separately.

It was clear that patients expressed more grief when another patient died than when they saw others who were very ill. Those who were concerned about their own illness were not necessarily more concerned or affected by witnessing others' illness. 22.2 per cent of comments on this item indicated sadness and concern. Male patients,

Table 5 Average anxiety and depression scores and patients' comments on their condition across diagnostic groups

	Degenerative N = 65	Infective N = 29	Neoplastic N = 21
Average anxiety score and range	0.5 (0–10)	1.5 (0–7.5)	2 (0–7)
Average depression score and range	1.25 (0–18)	1.75 (0–6)	1 (0–8)
Total comments on 'their own condition'	501	197	131
Negative comments on 'their own condition'	161	69	55
% of negative comments	32.1	35.0	42.0

N.B. Anxiety maximum score = 12   Depression maximum score = 24

on the whole, were more casual about seeing others who were very ill, whereas females, particularly females in the younger age group, were often extremely upset by this.

Being away from the family and work have been reported to be distressing by Cartwright (1964) and McGhee (1961). In this study 44 per cent of all comments on being away from the family reflected sadness and in the case of older patients this was often combined with worry about how their spouse could cope alone at home. In fact males of over 40 years made more negative comments than others on this subject (these results can be seen from Table 6).

Table 6 Patients' comments on being away from their family and work

	Males under 40	Males 40 and over	Females under 40	Females 40 and over
Total comments on being away from family	n = 47 288	n = 45 270	n = 46 350	n = 37 287
Number of negative comments	118	142	140	131
% of negative comments	41.0	52.6	40.0	45.6
Total comments on being away from work	n = 47 299	n = 26 215	n = 38 310	n = 20 102
Number of negative comments	88	79	84	22
% of negative comments	29.4	36.7	27.1	21.6

Being away from work affected 131 patients in this sample and 29.5 per cent of their comments were negative. These ranged from 'wondering what was going on without me', to 'being very bored without work' and 'missing my friends'. A reduction in income

Metabolic N = 31	Psychosomatic N = 7	Mechanical N = 14	Congenital N = 4	Allergic N = 11	Other N = 20
0.5	2	1.25	1.5	1.25	2
(0–5)	(0–10)	(0–4)	(0–3)	(0–3)	(0–7.5)
1	2	2	0.5	1.5	0.5
(0–7.5)	(0–20)	(0–4)	(0–4)	(0–9)	(0–11)
186	66	102	12	44	149
60	47	30	5	12	57
32.3	71.2	29.4	41.7	27.3	38.3

certainly affected many self-employed males and fear of actually losing their job affected many, particularly males over 40 years. Negative comments on these subjects were made sporadically throughout patients' stay.

Many patients commented that being in hospital was certainly not the best way to have a rest cure! Despite night sedation over a third (36.2 per cent) of all the nights spent in hospital by these patients were said to be disturbed. Although this may not mean that they lost a great deal of sleep 161 patients certainly felt as though they were not rested (two thirds of the sample were in the long open wards).

This is certainly not an original finding and nurses have obviously not been able to improve the situation since the survey results of the early 1960s (Cartwright, 1964; McGhee, 1961). Noise from other patients was blamed most frequently but proximity of one's bed to either a sluice or kitchen was shown to be a close second. Lights from these areas and constant traffic prevented sleep.

When comparing the type of night's rest between open wards or cubicles of 3 to 4 or single bed accommodation, it was clear that the cubicle patients had fewer disturbed nights. Those most susceptible to disturbed nights were either of high emotionality, younger females, or patients in the higher socio-economic classifications. There was a certain adjustment to night time in hospital. Over half the patients complained of having more disturbed nights at the beginning of their stay.

'The doctor's visit' was discussed because of its acknowledged importance to the patients. By far the majority of patients were appreciative and 'positive' in their remarks about their doctors. In all, only 12.8 per cent of responses about the daily visit of their ward doctor were negative in any way. About half these negative comments related to some undesirable or unwanted information they received from the doctor during their conversation. Only 5 per cent of comments were negative in a critical way. These concerned an apparent lack of attention from the doctor or disappointment in their treatment and were more frequently made at the end of the patients' stay in hospital. Patients were certainly displeased when doctors did not pay their expected daily visit.

In contrast, there were many more negative comments from patients after their consultant's round. 49 per cent of all comments from both hospitals' samples reflected disapproval or discouragement after the round. Patients often felt that they did not know what had been decided, that they had not been included in the conversation or were embarrassed at having been the centre of so many doctors' attention. Younger males were particularly negative, as were those categorised as highly emotional and those in the degenerative and infective categories.

Despite these negative comments, anxiety scores for the round days from patients who had been seen by the consultant and his team were no higher than their average scores. This may have been due to the short-lived emotional reactions caused by the round or because many comments tended to be critical rather than an expression of distress.

From this study it was clear that particular types of patients report most anxiety and depression during their stay in hospital. For example, patients with high emotionality scores on the EPI were those who reported strong negative emotions and who were likely to make most negative comments, while in hospital. These patients frequently responded to admission, to special tests, to doctor's rounds or to the weekends in hospital with strong feelings of anxiety and depression, whereas those who had low emotional predispositions would only report slight anxiety, even on quite stressful occasions. The distribution of these patients across personality groups is shown in Table 7.

or sex or more sophisticated ones such as career achievement.

Table 7 Patients reporting strong emotional reactions* during hospitalisation across EPI groups

	High emotionality n = 56	Medium emotionality n = 122	Low emotionality n = 24
Hospital 'A'	11	7	3
Hospital 'B'	9	5	2
% of total sample	9.9	5.9	2.5

*Those patients reporting anxiety score of 4 or more for at least a third of their stay or depression score of 6 or more for at least a third of their stay. Alternatively those who reported peaks of anxiety of 6 or more or of depression of 8 points or more at least twice during their stay.

Females under 40 years reported relatively frequent feelings of anxiety and depression. This is perhaps not surprising in the light of other evidence which points to the vulnerability of younger women who experience and express anxiety and depression in everyday life (Ayd, 1961). However, these findings may also be a function of events occurring in the female wards. These were usually busy and often full of elderly or seriously ill patients. In particular those who are admitted for investigations should be considered 'at risk'. Their scores were often elevated due to special tests and they were often really worried about the seriousness of their unknown complaint.

Lastly, those patients in the neoplastic and infective groups were subject to strong emotional reactions even though these were fairly short lived in the case of the infective group. It is suggested, however, that patients who are being investigated or are in the early stages of a malignant disease in medical wards may well be more emotionally reactive than those who know of their condition and have adjusted to it.

These findings lead to certain statements that could be helpful in identifying groups of patients who are 'at risk' of extreme emotional reactions while in hospital.

In summary, the following patients reported higher levels of anxiety and depression throughout their stay:

1. Females under 40 years.
2. Patients admitted for investigation.
3. Those suffering from neoplastic, infective or unknown disorders.
4. Patients who are generally prone to feelings of anxiety and depression, as indicated by a personality inventory.

A combination of these factors in any one patient should alert hospital staff who want to prevent distress. Despite the self-report nature of all these data, which should if possible be verified by replication, nurses, in particular, may like to observe patients more closely in order to assess their feelings and to direct their psychological care to those who are likely to need it especially at times of admission to the ward or going for a special test.

CONCLUSION

It seems clear that there are several aspects of hospitalisation which cause distress to patients, but that certain patients are more likely to become distressed by these. Poor communications between staff and patients is one subject which is mentioned frequently and Cartwright (1964) considered that this problem became graver in the larger hospitals. The lack of a 'personal touch' and a systematic supply of information has been a source of comment in most of the surveys in the last twenty years. This may account for much unnecessary stress in patients and methods of preventing this will be discussed in the concluding Chapter.

This complex subject is in need of further research which can explain how staff can alleviate the distressing aspects of hospital life, build on previous work identifying those patients who are in particular need of psychological support and demonstrate ways for implementing strategies which will humanise hospitals.

5

The experience of a special test

In the studies discussed in Chapter 4, it was found that a special diagnostic test, which involves either a patient going to another department or a specialist coming to the ward to carry out a procedure, was a very stressful experience for general-ward patients. In the longitudinal study described (Wilson-Barnett and Carrigy, 1978) the patients reported significantly more anxiety on 'special test' days than others. 78 per cent of all patients' comments about special tests were negative. In some way these reflected anxiety over what would happen and how much discomfort would be experienced. The degree of anxiety reported was not always shown to be related to the personality factors of emotionality and reactions were often not related to the amount of discomfort or the seriousness of the test. Age and sex variables also had little influence on the reactions, in that most female and male patients, of all ages, felt negative or anxious in some way.

As previously discussed, many studies have indicated that the amount of information patients said they were given by staff was inadequate. In further research information given to patients before special diagnostic tests was assessed in particular to see if there was any relation between giving information and reports or signs of patient anxiety and discomfort. In order to appreciate the work in this field it is useful to outline the main aims, designs and difficulties in conducting these experiments. Abdellah and Levine (1965) discuss this in full with relation to research in nursing and patient care.

One purpose of doing experiments is to try to understand and explain a particular situation and the relationship between two or more variables in bringing about that situation. Fundamentally, it may be described as what happens to A when B occurs; but to examine this event B must be a constant and A must be measurable. What is attempted in an experiment is, therefore, to control all other variables that may influence the interaction of A and B. The independent or introduced factor (i.e., B) is exposed to the experimental situation (i.e., A) in a standard way and the effect it has on A is measured. The classical way of assessing whether the independent variable (B) affects a change in the dependent (A) variable is by comparing two groups, one of which is subjected to the experimental or independent variable (B) and the other which is not.

However, the real world is a complex environment with 'complex' subjects and there are unwanted influences which may distort the purity of the ideal experiment. With human subjects there are often many intrinsic or organismic variables which alter responses and there are also many organisational variables which affect the independent experimental factors. Various attempts can be made to limit unwanted or extraneous influences. Control of the environment in applied experiments is usually very difficult so the study is designed for subjects who seem to be affected by similar environmental factors. Control of the effects of intrinsic variables is also problematic but again researchers can sometimes achieve a similar distribution of relevant factors between control and experimental groups. Thus subjects are assigned to each group by matching such items as age and sex or, if the number of subjects is large enough, by randomisation of the distribution of intrinsic variables in the experimental and control groups.

For research in the health care field there are advantages and disadvantages to using the experimental approach. Explanations for various effects may be provided, the results are intended to be free of contaminating influences, and variables can be manipulated to provide more and different information. However, with human beings in a 'complex' situation, the variables are often ill-defined and therefore often not measurable (such as degree of pain experienced or the success of rehabilitation). With human subjects some experiments are not ethically justifiable. Subjects must be given an outline of the study purpose, which may alter their behaviour in the research situation. It is usually impossible to standardise many of the organisational influences in health care. The effects of some changes or independent factors are seen only after quite a lengthy period of time, giving more opportunity for other changes to have influenced the dependent variable. Lastly, most behaviour is over-determined or is multifactorial in production so that a direct cause and effect relationship is undetectable.

With these qualifications in mind one can assess experiments and their contributions more accurately with regard to the effects of special procedures in hospital. An early clinical experiment by Meyers (1964) is a good example of an attempt to manipulate the variables in an experimentally created stressful situation which resembled a diagnostic test. She aimed to test the 'effects of three different conditions of communication on the impact and resulting cognitive structuring of an unfamiliar and moderately stressful situation'. The investigator approached patients with a tray containing a dry test tube, one containing warm water, gauze swabs, applicator sticks and a metal container. She got the patients into bed, uncovered the inner aspect of the arm and then swabbed an area with the water, the area was covered with gauze and then at 15-second intervals this was lifted and the area inspected. After one minute the area was dried and the materials placed in the container.

With the sample of 72 hospitalised patients divided into three groups Meyers enacted three types of communication during this procedure. The first explained exactly what she was going to do – she explained that the water was a solution used to test for allergy – a routine procedure done on all patients. The second group had no communication from the researcher except, 'just a minute'. The third group were subject to irrelevent conversation.

Following this procedure there was a post experimental inverview with each patient assessing recall of items on the tray and the procedure adopted. The degree of the patient's 'tension' was assessed by whether they mentioned the words 'blood' or 'needle'. They scored one point if they did mention them and none if not. The third system of rating measured their degree of talkativeness, and whether there was a degree of 'overestimation' or 'underestimation' in their recall of the procedure.

Findings from this study claimed to show that significantly more patients recalled details accurately in the explanation groups than the other two. More of the patients who did not receive explanation mentioned 'blood' or 'needle' and no differences were found on the over- and underestimation scores. Meyers concluded that 'less tension is created when the patient is given information upon which he can structure the event of impending stress'.

There are three areas which can usefully be discussed in assessing this early attempt to apply experimental principles to assessing a 'pseudo clinical' situation. The first is the possible contamination of measures by the researcher's knowledge of the experimental group of each subject. That is, the testing was not 'blind' and interpretation of the patients' behaviour may have been biased by knowledge of their experimental group and the desire for a particular outcome. The second is the crudity of the 'fear' measure of whether or not needles or blood were mentioned. There is no previous evidence demonstrating that a positive correlation exists between fear and mention of needles or blood. The third concerns the conclusion that fear was associated with poor recall. This relates to the previous point that fear had not been adequately demonstrated so Meyers cannot conclude that it was associated with recall. Perhaps one should also mention that, although the procedure was not physically harmful, some may argue it did go beyond the bounds of ethical standards in that the explanation included an untruth, that all patients had this test for allergy.

Later experiments in the area of explanation and patients' or subjects' reactions to fears may well have benefitted from refining Meyers' type of methods. For instance, Johnson and Rice (1974) hypothesised that those who had accurate expectations of a painful experience would actually report less pain and distress than those who did not. They tested this on 52 males in a laboratory by assessing the experience of ischaemic pain induced by a sphygmomanometer cuff being inflated to 250 (mmHg). They divided the sample into 4 groups with the following conditions:

1. A description of sensations unlikely to occur with ischaemic pain.
2. A description of only two of the sensations the subject could expect to experience.
3. A description of all the typical sensations experienced.
4. A description of the procedure void of sensations.

Two researchers were involved in this study. One gave the explanation and the other performed the inflation of the cuff and put on the tape which instructed how the subject should do a fist clenching series of exercises necessary to induce pain. Three stages occurred for each subject: the cuff was inflated three times and pain was rated each time. After each inflation a mood adjective check list was completed which measured the degree of well-being, fear, anger, helplessness, and depression.

An analysis of variance test was then undertaken to assess differences between distress and pain-rating in the four groups. The partial-sensory and the full-sensory informed subjects had lower scores on the distress rating than non-informed and procedurally informed. Those who were fully informed of sensations reported less physical sensation, overall, than others. They concluded: 'accurate expectations about sensations reduce emotional reactions to painful stimuli when the perception of the degree of danger in the situation is held constant'.

This study provides an example of a laboratory study, well controlled with blind testing. One can always be critical of applying the results of these studies to the clinical setting. Work by Johnson and colleagues, discussed below, forestalls this.

Johnson, Kirchhoff and Endress (1975) conducted an experiment in the same department, whereby children due for plaster of paris cast removal were assigned to one of three information groups:

1. Sensory information, describing sensory experience during cast removal.
2. Procedure information, describing steps of the experience.
3. Control group with no information.

Groups 1 and 2 listened to taped information prior to the cast removal and all three groups were observed and rated according to their behaviour. Group 1 had the lowest distress rating, and Group 2 rating was intermediate and Group 3 had a significantly higher distress score.

Another experimental study by Johnson, Morrissey and Leventhal (1973) is also of direct relevance to this subject. A sample of patients due for endoscopic (gastroscope) examination were divided into three groups. One group heard a taped passage which described the sensations most people experience. A second heard a preparatory message which gave an objective description of the procedure. The third group (the control group) heard no message. Messages were recorded on tape and accompanied by photographs. The sample included 99 in- and out-patients. Behavioural indicators of distress and fear were recorded (blind) during the examination by a third researcher. Indicators included the dose of diazepam (Valium) required by the patient in order to tolerate the procedure; heart-rate changes during the examination; hand and arm movements indicating tension during tube passage, gagging and restlessness. The results showed that controls required significantly more Valium than the other two groups and the tension scores for the sensation group were significantly lower than for both the control and procedure group. Johnson et al conclude that the nearer the anticipated experience is to reality, the lower the resulting anxiety or tension levels. Once more this is a good example of controlled clinical research.

A more recent study by Hoare and Hawkins (1976) also aimed to assess the reactions of patients to endoscopy. They compared 200 patients' responses by whether they had Valium given intravenously as a pre-operative sedation or not. Unsedated patients were found to rate the experience as more unpleasant and were worried about a repeat examination and more of them failed to tolerate the experience. A further 100 patients who were selected as more suitable to withstand the procedure without sedation were also studied. There was no difference between this group and the sedated group. Women of all ages were said to be less able to tolerate endoscopy unsedated, as were men under 40 years.

Although the sample was very adequate for this study the initial selection was not random and the findings relied mostly on data collected by questionnaire given long after the event. This, of course, would rely on memory which may easily be affected by both intrinsic and extrinsic factors. Although this study did not assess the effect of discussion with patients prior to gastroscopy the author's conclusion suggested this was a beneficial preparation. The conclusion here was, therefore, not related to research findings.

The research reviewed above has usually focused on the most stressful procedures for hospital patients. Other studies suggest, however, that more routine tests may be just as stressful for patients experiencing them for the first time.

Findings from an exploratory interview study, discussed above, (Wilson-Barnett, 1976) prompted further research. One of the items discussed with patients in that study concerned their reaction to X-rays. Forty-four of the 200 medical-ward patients interviewed had experienced either a barium meal or enema and 38 said they found it was either uncomfortable or unpleasant, or evoked anxiety.

In addition to these findings an interview survey by Wild and Evans (1968) with patients referred for barium, gall bladder and pyelographic examinations demonstrated that a large number were fearful of these tests. Of the 282 who were asked about prior knowledge of the test 259 had been given no authoritative information. Of these 282 patients 139 would have liked more information by either a leaflet or a personal talk and 70 of them felt that prior knowledge would have actually altered their reaction.

In view of all these findings it was decided to test patients' emotional responses to these procedures and assess the effect of giving a prior, explicit description of the procedure on these responses, to see if this might reduce anxiety and give guidance for future hospital practice (Wilson-Barnett, 1978). Explanation was, therefore, used as the independent variable in an experimental study of patients' emotions before and during a barium meal or enema. Specifically, the experiment attempted to answer two questions:

1. To what extent do patients experience negative emotions immediately prior to and during barium X-rays?
2. Does explanation of a barium X-ray lessen the amount of negative emotional reaction felt prior to and during the procedure?

Patients scheduled for either a barium meal or enema who had not previously experienced such an investigation were included in the experiment. These patients were assigned alternately to either an experimental or a control group. The experimental group received a written and verbal explanation of the investigation they were to have the next morning. The explanations were based on information gained from a week's observation in the X-ray screening rooms during barium X-rays and on patients' comments about these procedures. Additional details about preparation for X-rays were also obtained from radiographers and radiologists. Patients' comments and descriptions about the procedures were noted and vocabulary used by them was incorporated in the explanation sheet and verbal explanation. The verbal explanation was standard and took approximately five minutes. Patients' questions were answered at any time during this explanation. The sheet was given to them to read and keep. The control group did not receive this information. The 'interactor' visited them for the same time as the explanation took and asked how they were getting on in hospital. This led to unsystematic interaction. In every other aspect the control subjects were treated like the experimental group.

Two researchers were necessary for the 'cross-over' design of the experiment. For half of the sample, one person would 'test' while the other interacted or gave the explanation; for the other half they would switch roles. This enabled the testing to be done without awareness of the subject's experimental condition (i.e., blind). It also enabled results to be compared to assess the effects of the person explaining on patients' anxiety levels. If both researchers had the same beneficial effect this would obviously give more confidence in applying the practice of explanation beyond this research study.

On the day prior to X-ray the tester would consult the list of patients due for barium studies in the X-ray department. Every patient scheduled for barium X-ray who had not experienced that specific procedure before was included in the experiment. The tester would then visit all these patients to ascertain whether they fitted the sample criteria and if so to request their help in the research. The study was described to them as a nursing project designed to discover how patients feel about such X-rays.

Research instruments used in this study included a mood adjective check list, describing anxiety, depression and three other factors. It contained 24 adjectives, most of which were used to mask the anxiety words. It was used as a state measure, that is to report present feelings and was applied on four occasions. The EPI (Eysenck and Eysenck, 1964) was also used, but only once as it is a trait test of emotionality and extroversion. This was used to compare experimental and control groups for any differences and to provide information on the reactions of highly emotional subjects as compared to low 'N' scorers.

Testing with the mood adjective check list was undertaken on four occasions:

1. At the initial visit to patients at approximately 3 p.m. on the afternoon prior to X-ray. This was known as the baseline measurement.
2. After the interactor's visit at approximately 5 p.m.
3. Half an hour before X-ray, in the ward.
4. Within half an hour after the X-ray to describe feelings during the X-ray.

In addition, patients completed the EPI after the tester's first visit and this was collected on a subsequent visit.

In order to examine the null hypothesis that anxiety was not significantly less in the experimental group during and prior to the barium X-rays it was necessary to compare the anxiety scores of the controls with the experimental group in each of the four stages of mood rating.

The baseline score 1 for anxiety and depression were first compared. It was necessary to establish that no differences existed between these initial scores before statistical testing of the three succeeding stages for differences between experimental and control conditions.

The EPI 'N' score was then compared with the baseline score to indicate if baseline scores were related to patients' usual level of emotionality. The Spearman rank order correlation was used. Patients were also divided into 'high', 'medium' and 'low' emotionality groups. Within these groups experimental and control groups were compared. This served to show whether different responses to both X-ray and to explanation existed within these groups.

Prior to doing the main study a brief pilot study was carried out on twenty patients having a barium meal and twenty having a barium enema. This was done to test the practicality and efficacy of the method.

The two histograms (below) show the results of the main study. It can be seen that some degree of anxiety was reported in both meal and enema samples. The degree of anxiety evoked by enema is greater than that during a barium meal. The effect of explanation in reducing anxiety was most clearly demonstrated during the barium enema where comparisons with the Mann Whitney U tests were significantly different. The experimental group's anxiety scores were less during the barium meal, but this was not statistically significant. Although it also appeared that the experimental group were less anxious prior to enema this was only a trend which was not statistically significant.

This and other related research suggests that explanation reduces anxiety if it is given prior to a stressful episode. Barium meals did not evoke such high levels of anxiety for many subjects as enemata did. This may be explained by the fact that we are a tablet-taking nation and oral preparations are more commonplace and therefore less stressful than rectal administrations. Certainly the barium enema was considered more uncomfortable and embarrassing by both radiographers and the patients.

When scores were analysed and compared according to emotionality trait categories, results in all three groups were similar; that is, explanation was associated with reduced anxiety levels for all three experimental groups as compared to controls. However, there was a positive correlation between emotionality trait scores and the state anxiety scores at each stage of the experiment.

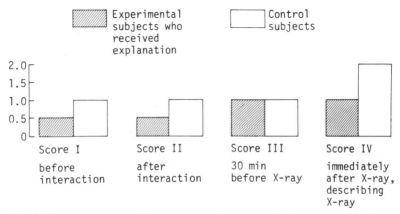

Fig. 3 Histogram representing average anxiety scores for barium meal patients. N = 58.

The assumption that a barium meal or enema is a standard procedure and that it has uniform effects and sensations for each patient can be criticised. During the week's observation and the pilot study the researcher attempted to assess whether certain physical disorders were associated with a more unpleasant procedure. For instance, inflammation of the bowel and anus may make a barium enema very unpleasant and painful. Four patients with colitis were interviewed and varying reports of their enema were given. This seemed to correspond to their personality factors rather than their physical condition, as suggested in this study. As it is so difficult to isolate pain reactions from anxiety responses it was decided to assume that a random allocation of patients into control and experimental groups would result in a fairly even distribution of patients with inflammatory or stenotic conditions.

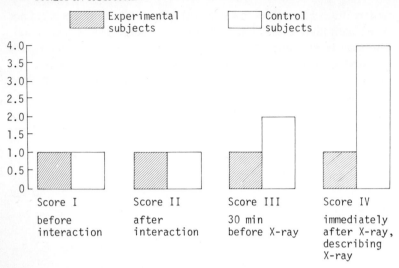

Fig. 4 Histogram representing average anxiety scores for barium enema patients. N = 70.

CONCLUSION

Some of the basic principles of applying experimental research to assessing aspects of care have been outlined and their application noted in studies. These studies provide a clear message for staff that providing information to patients is associated with reduced anxiety. In that the literature reviewed in Chapter 1 indicated the harmful nature of anxiety both on illness and recovery, it is obvious that nurses, doctors and others should reduce anxiety where possible. However, there is a problem in that, although supplying information is associated with reduced anxiety, some studies (e.g., Andrew, 1967) show that not much information is actually remembered by patients. For instance Ley and Spelman (1967) reported a study on out-patients' recall and found only 43.5 per cent of them remembered instructions given to them. The largest proportion, 86.4 per cent recalled their diagnosis but less than a quarter remembered all they were told. Clearly, before giving information the professional person needs to assess the type of interaction that will be most easily understood and appreciated by the patient.

6

Surgery – patients' reactions

The last Chapter discussed patients' reactions to special tests, the most frequently occurring stressful event in general medical wards. In surgical wards the more obviously stressful event is the surgical operation. There is now considerable research evidence that patients awaiting surgery experience negative emotions. In particular, they are fearful 'of the unknown' and the experience of pain post-operatively. In this section the aspects of surgery which evoke fear, the personality factors which affect responses to surgery and recovery and the research which has tested effects of information giving and taught coping methods, will be reviewed.

In a small study Carnevali (1966) explored patients' fears about pending surgery and compared these to their nurses' opinions on their patients' feelings. She found that out of 81 patients only 7 had absolutely no concerns. By asking 12 open questions she found two major areas of concern. The first was the degree of pain and discomfort they would have to suffer. The second was the fear of what might happen to them. The latter arose because of their unfamiliarity with surgical procedures and the content of their fear was, therefore, imagined or fantasised. Patients worried about themselves, about being 'cut', about dying, about change in their appearance and body and about losing control of their bodily functions and consciousness.

When comparing the patients' responses to the nurses' responses, nurses, on the whole, underemphasised how much the fear of pain affected their patients. They were more accurate, however, in their assessments of how the elements of the unknown impinged on them. Nurses reported that they helped patients by supplying information to alleviate fears, whereas patients reported them as 'just being friendly'. Patients also mentioned two instances in which nurses increased their discomfort pre-operatively, one by inserting a naso-gastric tube before anaesthesia and secondly when they could be overheard in the operating theatre arguing over a technical matter.

There are many aspects pre- and post-operatively which could easily be seen as stressful. One of these, pre-operative starvation, was studied by Hamilton-Smith (1971). In particular she looked at the varying length of time that was recommended by anaesthetists and found that this ranged from 3 to 12 hours or more. In assessing whether this length of time affected patients' recovery she suggested that factors such as dehydration, hypoglycaemia, possible electrolyte imbalance and physical discomfort should be considered relevant factors.

Minckley (1974) exploring this further, studied patients who had a delayed wait for surgery and monitored physiological and psychological indices pre- and post-operatively. Thirty patients who were scheduled for timed surgery and had less time 'nil by mouth' were compared with 30 who were starved longer for an operation to occur 'some time' in the afternoon. All these patients were due for hip replacement procedures and their speed of recovery, the outcome criteria, was assessed on 17 measures. Baseline measures of stress were taken one day before surgery and repeated for 14 days postoperatively. These measures included pulse rate and volume, galvanic skin response and plethysmography of the finger (two physiological measures of stress). A mood adjective check list, similar to the one discussed previously, was also used daily. Recovery measures were specifically designed for these orthopaedic patients. They included deep breathing, coughing, blowing up a balloon, lifting the hips off the bed after 24 hours, absence of nausea, vomiting or fever and no difficulty in either micturition, defaecation or eating. Patients were expected to be able to dangle their legs over the side of the bed on the fifth postoperative day and to sit in a chair on the sixth for 15 to 30 minutes, to use a walking frame on the seventh, to undertake special exercises by the tenth and also to use crutches on the tenth day. The results of this study demonstrated no significant differences between the rate of recovery between the two groups of patients. This suggests that the length of pre-operative starvation does not influence recovery. However, these results need to be qualified as routines for the rehabilitation activities of orthopaedic patients are dependent on the behaviour and attitudes of the staff as much as the progress or willingness of the patients. They are also not really suitable for general application to other specialities. As with other aspects of illness these results could also be related to personal patient factors, rather than environmental elements. In addition 30 patients in each group may have been insufficient to ensure an even distribution of certain intrinsic (personal) factors between the groups.

Personality factors have been shown in previous Chapters to relate to patients' reactions to events in hospital and research on surgical patients has produced findings indicating that emotional reactions, degrees of pain and patients' progress postoperatively are affected by certain dimensions of their personality.

Janis (1958) conducted interviews with patients undergoing surgery and made observations about levels of pre-operative anxiety and post-operative recovery. He considered that extreme anxiety experienced before operation heralded a stormy recovery. Similarly absence of any feelings of apprehension or normal fear was also not conducive to a smooth rehabilitation. The ideal state, he considered, was a realistic degree of anxiety which stimulated patients to cope with the situation. These patients needed to know what would happen to prevent unanticipated stress. They could only plan for events and sensations if anticipated events were realistic.

Related to this study, Johnson, Dabbs and Leventhal (1970) traced emotional reactions to see how predispositions would influence both physical recovery and patients' feelings. They studied emotional traits but also classified patients according to an internal–external dimension. 'Internal' people tend to believe that what happens to them is their responsibility and they have power to determine their fate. 'External' people, on the other hand, conceive that they are in the hands of fate which is, therefore, out of their control. Johnson *et al.* hypothesised that the internal people would attempt to seek information so that they themselves could manage the situation and attempt to cope with surgery. In that previous evidence had suggested that first-borns were more dependent on reassurance from others and were thought to be more sensitive to pain, the researchers also considered the position of the patient in the family.

They studied 62 patients who were scheduled either for cholecystectomy or hysterectomy. They requested that patients complete four questionnaires on the pre-operative evening and a mood adjective check list and a self report of their degree of pain, each morning from the first to the fifth postoperative day. From this study the authors concluded that the trait measures of emotionality were a good predictor of state anxiety scores before and after operation. The observations made by Janis were not confirmed. Similar levels of anxiety were found usually before and after operation and moderate, pre-operative anxiety was not necessarily conducive to the best post-operative recovery. 'Internals' were found to receive more analgesics and the first-born patients tended to stay in hospital longer than others, confirming part of their hypothesis.

A series of experimental studies has been done to assess the effects of giving information to patients pre-operatively. One of the first by Egbert, Battit, Welch and Bartlett (1964) aimed to test if a visit by an anaesthetist to explain about the types of pain, methods for pain relief and relaxation exercises would influence the patients' length of stay, consumption of analgesia and general progress. They found that the length of stay was shorter for those who were informed and also that they required fewer analgesics. Other studies have not always had the same results, although a recent project by Leigh, Walker and Janaganathan (1977) with a sample of 32 patients did confirm Egberts' findings. They used Speilberger's trait-state inventory for measuring anxiety before an explanatory visit by a member of the research team and then three hours after this. One group of twelve patients were given a verbal explanation of the anaesthetic, another group of twelve were given a written version of this explanation and a control group had no explanation. Anxiety levels of the first group were lower than the other two groups but the second group was also significantly less anxious than the controls. Unfortunately, interpretation of these findings is rendered impossible by the many relevant variables and the wide range of procedures. In addition, the experimental groups could easily gauge the hypothesis and report anxiety accordingly to please the anaesthetic team because members of the anaesthetic team carried out both the explanation and the testing.

Hayward's (1975) study included both male and female patients and measured anxiety factors, pain ratings, analgesia consumption, post-operative complications and length of stay. He hypothesised that experimental patients who had a comprehensive pre-operative explanation including anaesthetic and operative techniques, post-operative sensations, schedules and exercises, would be less anxious, have less pain and few complications. He found that experimentally informed patients required fewer analgesics over a defined post-operative period than others. Patients who were more anxious reported more pain and women were given more analgesics than men. An important finding from this study related to the fact that it was the nurses who were the ones who determined the amount of analgesia the patients received, how often and for how long post-operatively, rather than the patients or the doctors.

Another nursing research study used physiological parameters to measure the difference in stress levels between an informed group of surgical patients and their controls. Boore (1976) studied 60 patients scheduled for cholecystectomy. Prior to operation 30 of these patients were given an extensive account of their care and expected progress from the pre-operative day until discharge. They were also given the opportunity to ask questions. Boore stressed that the explanation included procedural and experiential details. Control patients received a non-explanatory interview by the researcher.

The parameters chosen to reflect physical and psychological stress were pulse, blood pressure, temperature and urinary catecholamines. The patients' feelings of wellbeing were also assessed daily. Boore found that informed patients had fewer infections post-operatively and had a significantly lower level of urinary catecholamines and other physiological and psychological indices of stress.

When reviewing pre-operative care of patients, Boore (1977) also shows how pre-operative sessions of informing patients about exercises were shown to reduce post-operative complications. For instance, deep breathing, coughing and bed exercises were found by Lindeman and Van Aernam (1971) to improve post-operative ventilatory function so reducing the length of stay and total amount of analgesics consumed.

The studies reviewed here suggest that pre-operative preparation including detailed explanations tend to effect a reduction in anxiety. However, certain personality factors, such as a high trait of emotionality may be a more powerful determinant of high levels of pre- and post-operative anxiety. A high level of pre-operative anxiety may prevent use of this information and interrupt any rehearsal of coping strategies. It is nevertheless interesting that, in a controlled trial, patients previously given information had a reduced anxiety level but could not recall the information (Andrew, 1967).

In all these studies a fairly standard explanation is given to patients. It may be that if the information and explanation was tailored to individual patients' requests and needs it could be even more effective. For instance, different levels of understanding and imagination probably require different modes of communication. But there is still a perpetual problem with the few patients who do not want to hear about their operation or treatment and use a defensive denial. Janis (1958) discussed this and considered that these patients who had not prepared themselves pre-operatively were poor post-operative risks. They refused to think about the discomfort and restrictions on return from operation and because they denied that this situation would exist became uncooperative and hostile. But Janis thought it was necessary to evoke a 'reasonable' amount of anxiety to encourage thoughts on how to cope with the threat of surgery. Denial in other situations has previously been considered in Chapter 2, where it was suggested that denial may represent an expression of anxiety. It remains a very debateable point as to whether staff should force the patient to accept certain undesirable facts about surgery and how far denial should be broken down.

The value of reducing anxiety pre- and post-operatively to adaptive levels is two-fold. Apart from helping the patient to be less distressed it is aimed at reducing biological stress processes, which have been demonstrated to interrupt tissue healing processes (see Ch. 1). Further work by Langer, Janis and Wolfer (1975) has attempted to evaluate counselling sessions for pre-operative patients based on Janis' earlier ideas. These sessions involved encouraging an optimistic reappraisal of anxiety-provoking events to build up hope and the ability to cope effectively with surgery. Patients were trained to think of positive consequences of surgery whenever they felt anxious. This method of cognitive reappraisal was found to reduce stress before and after an operation, as rated (blind) by nurses. Patients who received this counselling also required fewer sedatives and analgesics than a control group.

CONCLUSION

These studies indicate that patients in surgical wards benefit from explanation, as do those in medical wards. Lowered anxiety levels pre- and post-operatively have been shown, in some studies, to be associated with more rapid and straightforward recovery. This in turn seems to be effected by pre-operative explanation which helps patients to cope with surgery and post-operative events. The type of explanation and the staff most suited and able to give this will be discussed in the concluding Chapter.

7

Patients' reactions to intensive care units

Patients who need highly specialised and technical care are usually admitted to intensive care units (ICU). These units are either for immediately post-operative patients or those with serious trauma, respiratory, renal or cardiac disorders. The environment in such units is so different from the general ward and so dominated by the various machines required to monitor cardiac, respiratory or other vital functions that it is no surprise to find stress reactions among patients.

There are two main differences in the psychological reactions noted in surgical ICUs as compared with coronary care units (CCU). While in both many emotional and psychological problems are found, those in the CCU tend to be milder but of more influence for later complications, in contrast to the more bizarre and obvious ones in the ICU. These are usually short-lived and the surgical patient is often amnesic of these events. The ICU is also associated with an uncomfortable, painful time for the patient recovering from a major operation, whereas in the CCU, patients are not usually in pain and are mainly observed and reassured by the staff. The result, as pointed out by Baxter (1975) is that patients leaving the ICU are pleased to have improved beyond the need for the intensive care whereas coronary patients may become very insecure and anxious in an open medical ward with relatively few nurses and so many more patients.

INTENSIVE CARE UNITS

The incidence of psychological morbidity after surgery tends to increase in the more serious, lengthy forms of open heart surgery or other major operations. It has been estimated that between 38 and 70 per cent of patients in some ICUs suffer from extreme psychological symptoms (Baxter, 1975). These are usually said to be related to various organic changes during the major cardiac operations as well as the effects of the 'intensive care'. However, even organically-induced psychological states can be affected by environmental changes.

Melia (1977) discusses the problems in ICUs from both the staff and patients' viewpoints. She describes the elements which serve to disorientate the patients as:

1. Sleep deprivation, particularly in the early post-operative period.
2. Feelings of being chained to the bed by the drips, drains and leads.
3. The frequently unpleasant procedures such as suction, being ventilated and turned.
4. The continual presence of the staff.

These factors, she says, may easily precipitate the post-operative psychotic episodes and paranoid symptoms which have been described in, for example, open heart surgery patients. She described how Lawrie (an analytic chemist who recorded his experiences) felt in response to curare and respiratory ventilation. He had double vision and the impression that things were very near and large, the ceiling, for instance, seemed to be eighteen inches away. He also had unusually acute hearing and could hear what was being said by others much further away than usual. His worst memories were of being 'sucked' and thereby disconnected from the ventilator.

If one concludes that these sensations are experienced by many post-operative patients in the ICU it is not surprising that psychoses develop or are exacerbated. In Kornfield's (1969) study 38 per cent of post-operative cardiothoracic cases were said to become psychotic after three to four days. Symptoms included hallucinations, illusions, recent memory loss and paranoia. This was thought to relate to older age groups, evidence of organic brain damage and the length of time in surgery and on the cardio-pulmonary by-pass. Baxter (1975) says that this is a short-lived disturbance which settles after transfer from the unit and discusses how it is probably worsened by the ICU environment. As well as difficulties in sleeping, there is a sensory monotony produced by continually hissing oxygen tents and regularly flashing cardiac monitors. He likens this to sleep and sensory deprivation situations which are created experimentally and have been shown to lead to psychoses.

Baxter suggests that pre-operative explanations and interviews lower the incidence of delirium. This is in keeping with results reviewed in the last Chapter. He makes further suggestions; for instance, patients should also be talked to as soon as they return to the ICU, whether they appear to understand or not. They should also be orientated in time and place and reassured if they do hallucinate that this does often happen but that it will not influence or complicate their recovery. In some cases tranquillisers may be needed but the patient needs to understand what is happening to him and fit this alien environment into some sort of framework. He warns against platitudes (such as 'everything is fine' or 'don't worry') as they just become annoying and he advises that explanations should be simple and repeated when necessary. Although post-operative psychotic episodes are thought to be organic in origin, environmental factors can influence disorientated patients. Sensory deprivation from continual mechanical noises, the restrictions on mobility and minimal human contact of a familiar kind add to disorientation. Total darkness is also one of the most disorienting situations and although day–night sequence should be maintained, it is vital to allow dim night-lighting for these patients.

There have been studies to evaluate this type of normalising process in the environment of the ICU (Lazarus and Hagens, 1968). They have found that a pre-operative psychiatric interview and a revised recovery room procedure with more explanation and patient–staff interaction halves the incidence of post-cardiotomy delirium.

CORONARY CARE UNITS

The psychological problems associated with coronary care are more 'neurotic' than 'psychotic' and patients thus maintain awareness of their actions and feelings. Their emotional reactions, however, may have more effect on rehabilitation as they are of longer duration than those noted in the ICU patients. Lloyd (1977) has noted that anxiety is most intense at the time of maximal uncertainty about the outcome of the illness. In the case of myocardial infarction this is the first two days after the event. The danger of acute anxiety in some patients has been shown by the study of Vetter, Cay, Phillip and Strange (1977). They studied patients admitted with either a myocardial infarction or an acute ischaemic episode and found that those who were more anxious at the beginning of their illness were more likely to die. This may of course be associated with the severity of their illness. However, Baxter (1975) also asserts that there is 'much more direct evidence that in patients with myocardial infarction psychological upsets can have adverse physical affects and can in fact be fatal'. The explanation Vetter et al. gave for these results was that patients who died may have had premonitory symptoms such as angina and dyspnoea which increased their anxiety. As mentioned before, arrhythmias and further ischaemia have been shown to be related to a rise in catacholamine production (Carruthers, 1969) and increased coagulability of the blood. It is therefore important to reduce anxiety to prevent further cardiac damage.

Anxiety, however, is not the only reaction noted in these patients. Hackett, Cassem and Wishnie (1968) found that while 80 per cent of the coronary patients had symptoms of anxiety, 60 per cent were depressed and 16 per cent were agitated. Wynn (1967) also found that 50 per cent of coronary patients suffered from emotional distress, including depression, which led to psychological invalidism for a long time after their infarction.

Nagle, Gangola and Picton Robinson (1971) investigated the relationship between events in a CCU and rehabilitation. They studied 115 patients who had been working at the time of their coronary and found that about half of these patients did not return to work within a year of their discharge from hospital. Most importantly they found that invalidism was not related to physical incapacity in a majority of cases but more to their emotional reactions to their illness and fears of a relapse. They reported that 31 per cent of these patients experienced inadequate explanation and reassurance while in hospital. Other studies have found similar results, including those of Goble, Adey and Bullen (1963). While in hospital some patients were not allowed to move for several days and felt this to be the 'deathbed treatment'. More recently since more rapid mobilisation the risks of over-dependency leading to demoralisation have been reduced but a later study by Wishnie, Hackett and Cassem (1971) found that 9 out of 24 patients did not return to work because of psychological problems. They advise that patients would be helped by a more systematic plan of explanation and information giving from staff.

The psychiatrist's assistance was discussed by Freedman, Kaplan and Sadock (1975) and was said to reduce mortality rates in at least one study mentioned by them. They suggest the following approach to these problems in a CCU: '. . . proper use of tranquillisers and night time sedation, careful and detailed explanations of the significance of myocardial infarction and the attending psychological stresses, environmental manipulation, bolstering of optimism and confrontation of inappropriate behaviour'. They also suggest that there is much room for improved psychological support from nurses in such units, as one study showed that they spent only 1 per cent of their time talking to patients.

Baxter (1975) recommended that support in hospital should include some indication of when discharge from the unit is likely and commented that in some cases this is done quickly to make room for an admission. A nurse should then go with the patient to the general ward to confer with the staff about his special needs and should return to visit him each day to discuss plans and any queries he may have. The same physician throughout should be responsible for the patient to avoid interruptions in communications and therapy.

A plan for treatment and expected rehabilitation while in hospital can be written in a booklet as evaluated by Rahe (1975) and should include every aspect of life. This can be used as a focus of conversation and exploration when necessary. He also evaluated group sessions for coronary patients, where progress and fears were discussed and patients reported great comfort from this support for a long time after their discharge.

Results such as these suggest the same relationship between anxiety and lack of knowledge mentioned in the two previous Chapters is relevant to the recommendations for care of coronary patients. The presence of another person at time of stress (see Ch. 1) is also pertinent for each patient in a CCU. Nurses and others in the unit may be able to prevent stress reactions by their presence and willingness to be friendly and reassure the patient. This in turn may influence morbidity and mortality.

THE RENAL DIALYSIS UNIT AND MAINTENANCE DIALYSIS

Many of the stresses present in the coronary and surgical ICU exist for staff and patients in the renal dialysis units. Studies have highlighted the emotional problems of patients with kidney failure, maintained on dialysis. Kaplan De Nour (1970) reported the psychotherapeutic experience with twelve patients dependent on haemodialysis. The main sources of stress were seen as loss or threatened loss of body functions, dependency on machines, threat of death, inability to plan for the future and the frustration of drives, especially agressive ones. Neary (1976), in his review of data from dialysis units, confirmed that these areas of stress were usually mentioned. He suggested that depression was the most common reaction to renal failure but anxiety and irritability occurred in at least a third of chronic ureamics. Roger (1975) particularly mentioned how hard it was for nurses to cope with dying patients and for the patients to accept the inevitability of deterioration in health. He recommended that optimism was useful in the early days of kidney failure, that patients should have regular social contact and that defence mechanisms, such as denial and isolation, should be actively discouraged.

In a detailed account of patients' adjustment to outside life on maintenance dialysis Abram (1969) outlined four major phases. The first coincides with the ureamic syndrome characterised by fatigue apathy, drowsiness, an inability to concentrate and depression. The second stage occurs after dialysis was commenced, in which apathy lessens and gives rise to transient anxiety. Three weeks to three months after this the third stage of convalescence begins when the patient has to face reality. Depression is very likely to occur during this phase and Abram says that most patients do, in fact, consider suicide at this time. During the fourth stage there was a struggle for normality with return to work and usually after a year or so most people regain a positive will to live.

In a study to assess the quality of life for patients maintained on haemodialysis, 18 patients were interviewed by Levy and Wynbrandt (1975). It was found that over half the patients suffered a deterioration in their income and family life. This was also accompanied by a diminished frequency of sexual activity. Women were found to adjust more successfully and this was considered to be a result of their more flexible responsibilities in housekeeping. In contrast, over half the males were unable to return to full-time employment which inevitably led to a poor quality of life. The main factor which was said to contribute to adjustment to maintenance haemodialysis was a good supporting relationship with family and close friends.

Family members were interviewed to obtain their reactions to this maintenance treatment by Friedman, Goodwin and Chaudry (1970). With a small sample of 20 relatives they found that although family relationships had not deteriorated a large proportion mentioned the difficulties of maintaining outside activities of work or school due to the patient's diminished physical endurance. Eighteen of the relatives mentioned that they had noticed periodic depression in the patients and in the unmarried patients this was related to the difficulties of maintaining a satisfying social life.

In order to help patients adjust both to the process of haemodialysis in hospital or at home and to life maintained by this method psychotherapy has sometimes been given. Kaplan De Nour (1970) considers that most people agree that this has a place in these patients' management. Programmes are usually geared to encouraging independence by gaining confidence from gradually undertaking tasks such as travelling or clot extraction. Although some patients benefit more than others from psychotherapy it is said to help most to discuss their problems. Kaplan De Nour stresses that sympathy alone makes them more dependent and this should always be combined with encouragement and suggestions for positive coping behaviour.

THE NURSING STAFF

A different aspect of psychological reactions connected with intensive care units is the problem encountered by the staff themselves.

Nursing on these units involves different stresses but all situations require facing severe illness and frequent death. The deaths may be seen as failures where the *raison d'être* of the unit is saving lives. This dichotomy is often hard to accept. Frequently life and death decisions have to be taken by nurses often with little medical backing, such as responding immediately to the emergency of a cardiac arrest or haemorrhage. Melia (1977) sees all this as a paradox when nurses are forced to accept the hopeless case but will have to care for them in a curing atmosphere. Other stresses involve an initial adjustment to machines, repetitive routines, such as quarter-hourly observations, which will not really allow time for over-all care or assessments, a constant overload of work and a lack of gratification from patients. Because of the specialised nature of the work and added responsibilities for initiating emergency procedures the support system is not as effective as usual. Senior administrative staff are not so involved and relatives are often so anxious that they vent their feelings by criticising staff. In addition to all this, junior medical staff often work on a unit for a short period of time, while the nurses are there permanently and often resent these doctors requesting alterations in usual treatments or procedures.

The role of the psychiatrist in supporting staff has been discussed by Baxter (1975). He explains that staff's feelings of anxiety, fear and guilt can be beneficially explored when a psychiatrist is attached to the unit. Running regular meetings can serve to discuss any problematic incidents, thereby reducing tension. He also suggests that meetings may give junior staff a much needed opportunity to air their views. However, he does comment that these meetings should arise from a genuine wish on the part of the staff themselves. In fact, psychiatric involvement, either by a psychiatrist or by a psychologically trained nurse on intensive care units of all varieties is now becoming commonplace, both with a view to helping patients and also to helping staff through periods of stress. Evaluation of such support is underway. It is hoped that by such procedures wastage of staff, highly trained, may be arrested and the excessive turnover on these units relieved. Another possible way of helping was mentioned by Baxter (1975) who suggests a measure of over-staffing, and more rest-breaks for staff on such units.

Staff, as well as coping with their own feelings, must learn to recognise stress in their patients and in their patients' relatives. Although this is of course the case in general wards, it is perhaps even more important in the ICU setting. The nurses are often left to give news to relatives as they can establish relationships during the patients' stay in the unit. Of course, this puts an added strain on the unit staff since relatives may react with hostility during their grief and transfer their own anxieties to the staff. Melia (1977) discusses how relatives should be reassured as much as possible to prevent such anxiety being transferred either to staff or back to the patient.

CONCLUSION

It is, therefore, evident that there is a high risk of psychological morbidity for patients but also for staff in intensive care situations. The adverse effects of such reactions as anxiety and depression on health have been outlined and the abilities of staff to reduce it are suggested. Awareness of this may motivate staff to give more attention to psychological support for patients during their stay with the hope that they can be more fully rehabilitated in the future.

8

Patients' reactions to medications

Although many patients expect to be given a prescription when they visit their doctor, up to half of them fail to take their medications according to directions. From the abundance of documentation on this subject it appears to be a very important issue in health care. However, there is a paucity of hard facts predicting which patients are likely to be 'non-adherent' or 'non-compliant'.

An equally significant phenomenon related to patients' reactions to their medications is that of 'the placebo response'. This is said to occur when positive improvement in symptoms results from the administration of pharmacologically inert substances. Not only is this reaction important clinically, but it makes assessment of various active therapeutic agents difficult since patients are reacting to being given drugs rather than the active bio-chemical effects of the compounds. These two issues will now be discussed.

ADHERENCE TO MEDICATION

Despite actively seeking help and apparent reliance on medications many patients do not adhere to their doctors' prescriptions. To quote Rachman and Philips (1975) 'Doctors most commonly express discontent about the failure of their patients to carry out the advice or treatment recommended'.

Non-adherence to treatment regimes has become a focus of much attention and research, not only because of the possible dangers to patients who fail to take drugs but also because of the accumulation of potentially harmful drugs in many of their homes. It may be defined as failure to follow treatment schedules suggested, which includes errors of omission, purpose, dosage or timing and sequence. Blackwell (1976) also discusses over-dosage and taking additional medications which are not prescribed.

Failure to take medications as prescribed is a very complex reaction, apparently unrelated to any one type of illness, personality or social situation. However, there is agreement that it is a very prevalent problem and studies usually find that between 25 and 50 per cent of patients are non-adherent to some degree.

DETECTION OF NON-ADHERENCE

Marston (1970) describes how little consistency there is among researchers' indices of non-adherence and thereby a lack of comparability between studies. Obtaining a reliable measure seems very difficult. Merely asking the patient if they are taking their medications is notoriously unreliable. Measuring blood levels at a clinic visit may only indicate temporary or single dose consumption if traces are found.

The detection of a drug in the urine may denote some adherence but may not give an accurate picture of adherence. Urinary analysis may also falsify how many doses are taken regularly. Other methods for detecting non-adherence are also unsatisfactory. Patients may be reluctant to admit to non-adherence if asked and if their pill bottles are brought to the surgery these too may belie how many have been consumed. Patients often take a dose before they visit the doctor, to ease their conscience. Thus, if patients realise they may be questioned they may become temporarily adherent. As Marston mentions non-adherence is found to be higher at times of unannounced visits by the doctor.

FACTORS INFLUENCING NON-ADHERENCE

The rate of non-adherence is said to be highest among out-patients and lowest among in-patients. For instance Ley, Bradshaw and Eaves (1973) mentioned a previous study in which 48.7 per cent of out-patients failed to take antibiotics and 37.5 per cent of tuberculosis out-patients failed to take their drugs. Other studies on out-patients have found that even when patients attempt to adhere, up to 30 per cent may be taking the wrong drug at the wrong time. One factor with infectious diseases is the apparently quick relief of symptoms with chemotherapy and in common with many findings, a cessation of symptoms is related to a discontinuation of drug taking.

Even in hospital adherence is not total. As Roth and Berger (1960) found, hospitalised patients with gastro-intestinal ulceration who were told how much antacid to take throughout the day and were supplied with a sufficient quantity, only took 50 per cent of what was recommended.

It would appear that staff supervision of medication has a positive effect. Blackwell's (1976) review showed that adherence rates drop when staff supervision is reduced. The relative lack of supervision at home, after hospital care was thought to be a major factor. For instance, in a study of diabetics' adherence to insulin and diet regime at home, it was found that 80 per cent of the patients failed to administer their insulin in an acceptable manner, 50 per cent tested their urine in a way which would distort results and 73 per cent had unacceptable meals with unacceptable spacing of time (Watkins, Roberts, Williams, Martin and Coyle, 1967).

The types of illness predisposing to non-adherence have not been identified, but it seems fairly clear that chronic disorders are more likely to be related to patients' omissions than more acute, short lived illnesses. This is particularly likely to occur if symptoms do not return immediately after cessation of drug taking. Chronic disorders often require multiple drug therapy and complex regimes. This factor alone may confuse the patient and cause more inconvenience which again leads to non-adherence.

No one type of person is likely to become a non-adherent patient (Porter, 1969) as many risk factors have been mentioned but with low consensus in research findings. However, Blackwell suggests that non-adherence may be employed by some patients in an attempt to gain more support and supervision from other people. Both relatives and practitioners and other staff may unwittingly pay more attention to someone who is known to omit his treatment. Attempts through research to assess personality factors of non-adherers have been inconclusive. However, in view of the evidence which exists on the relationship of personality and reactions to illness it is likely that these factors also affect adherence. Predispositions of 'anxiety' and 'belief in personal control', which might be considered relevant were not found to be associated (Marston, 1970).

Other social and demographic factors have been studied with equally varied findings. In Marston's review (1970) sex and age factors were not found to be correlated with adherence in most research studies, although there is some indication that people of lower socio-economic status and those who are unmarried are more likely to be non-adherent. Patients who live alone have been found to be poor on adherence to medications and advice. However, if family members do not agree with treatment or are inconvenienced by collecting prescriptions this can also have a deleterious effect.

Lack of social support, complexity of regime and lack of faith in medications have all been related to higher rates of non-adherence. In addition Matthews (1975) suggests that patients who are depressed may be less likely to take drugs simply because 'they don't feel they are worth saving'.

One major factor found to affect adherence is the side effects of the medications prescribed. In general the presence of unpleasant symptoms due to medications increase the chance that patients will omit to take medications (Blackwell, 1976). For instance, in a drug trial by Porter (1969) comparing the effects of imipramine with a placebo, there was more non-adherence among those on imipramine, which is known to cause side effects. While slight dryness of the mouth was tolerated patients would not tolerate nausea or vomiting. In some cases, however, the presence of slight side effects may indicate to the patient that the drugs are actually 'working' and thereby promote adherence.

The situation and details of prescribing and administering medications has been shown to have a strong effect on whether patients take them as prescribed. As indicated in other Chapters a large proportion of patients find it difficult to understand what their doctor has said. In addition, it may be impossible for them to read the details of dosage from the labels on bottles. Obviously instructions have to be written legibly.

Extensive research into the communications and behaviour of the doctor when interviewing the patient has shown that this definitely affects adherence rates. For example, Korsch and Negrete (1972) found that patient satisfaction and adherence was related to the amount of sociable chit-chat that the doctors engaged in. Patients were more satisfied when their doctors were 'friendly' and chatted in this way. In this study most of the doctors thought they had been friendly whereas less than half the patients did! The importance of this aspect of care was confirmed by a study in a hypertensive clinic (Finnerty, Mattie and Finnerty, 1973). Non-adherence was reduced from 42 per cent to 8 per cent by streamlining appointments and offering a more personalised service.

The doctors manner and apparent friendliness is therefore related to their patients' satisfaction and subsequent co-operation in treatment. Difficulties arise when a doctor is faced with a patient who does not follow his advice. This is obviously frustrating and liable to make the doctor feel decidedly unfriendly. Matthews (1975) stresses how important it is that the doctor does not become angry. He should explore 'the possibilities of difficulty in taking the medication' rather than accuse patients of being unco-operative. The same approach obviously applies for nurses.

Ley and Spelman (1967) have shown that explanation and clear instructions from staff promotes adherence. However, there are problems. Many patients forget even carefully given instructions, and many doctors disagree that patients should know all about their medications (Ascione and Ravin, 1975). Poor communications are very likely if the doctor just assumes that instructions will be followed. Apart from this it has also been shown that doctors do tend to underestimate patients' knowledge and then give least information to those who are worst informed (see Rachman and Philips, 1975). A summary of the many factors influencing adherence is provided in the table below.

Table 8 A summary of factors which affect adherence (modified from Haynes and Sackett, (1976) *Compliance with Therapeutic Regimens*. Appendix 1, pp. 193–279. Baltimore: Johns Hopkins University press. © The Johns Hopkins University Press, 1976)

Positive	Negative
Patient considers disease as serious.	A complex regime of treatments which are socially inconvenient.
Minimal drug dosage (once a day if possible).	Treatments requiring major adjustment to life style.
A stable family and social life.	Undesirable side effects from medications.
Absence of side effects.	A chronic disease.
Patients' high level of satisfaction with treatment.	Living alone.
Close supervision from staff, monitoring of drug levels.	Lack of immediate recurrence of symptoms if medications are omitted.
Clear directions and information giving from doctors and nurses.	A lack of understanding of the importance of adherence or dangers of non-adherence.
Social and friendly interaction from staff.	Unclear labels on medications.
	Memory loss.

METHODS OF REDUCING NON-ADHERENCE

Davis (1968) found that adherence was associated with patient–doctor agreement, tension release and attempts to seek the patients' opinion about their illness and treatment. These elements should therefore be encouraged in treatment. In contrast he also found that rejection of the patient and requests to the doctor for information which were then not satisfied were related to non-adherence. These findings again point to the importance of establishing an easy flow of communication in this setting. Matthews (1975) reiterates this by saying that time spent talking to the patient will encourage adherence. He suggests assessing the patient's knowledge about his condition before commencing a regime and adjusting discussion accordingly. The patient should, when possible, join in the decision making process and then if the prescription is straightforward he will be more committed to it.

Joubert and Lasagna (1975) found that 92 per cent of patients wanted to know as much as possible about their medication. However

65 per cent did not actually want the responsibility for deciding how to organise their own drug administration. Any lack of motivation, therefore, has to be tackled in addition to the lack of retention of information. Blackwell (1976) suggests that patients should keep diaries to assess ease of adherence in their present life pattern and to enable detection of omissions and errors occurring. Adherence can then be monitored. This can be made less punitive by the doctor's open questions in regard to the patient's ease of management.

Although general education level has not been isolated as an influential factor in adherence most guidelines for advice include ways to impart clear, simple instructions to the patient. For instance, Ley and Spelman (1967) suggest this order of information:

1. Important things should come first, in logical sequence,
2. What is wrong with the patient.
3. What will be done for the patient.
4. What will then happen.
5. The complete treatment needed.
6. What the patient should do to help himself.

Blackwell (1976), in a similar format says there should be:

1. Clear goals for education.
2. Active involvement of the patient.
3. Multiple ways for imparting information and receiving feedback of the results.
4. Clarity, brevity and dialogue in the communication process.
5. Avoidance of anxiety, social distance and technical terminology.

These guides used systematically would probably help a patient to understand why he should comply.

One very obvious difficulty which Blackwell discusses is the transition from dependence in hospital to independence at home. Nurses check and administer medicines in hospital until the patient is discharged, they then expect him to take over responsibilities for administering his own drugs conscientiously. Convalescent patients should be prepared for discharge by an introduction into self-medication which will then, hopefully, be continued.

During the transition from patients taking medications given by nurses in hospital to self-administration at home, it may be helpful to involve relatives in discussions and explanations about drugs. They will then be able to remind the patient when they are due and perhaps encourage adherence during a chronic illness. Nurses in hospital often leave explanations about medications to the moment before discharge. It seems more sensible, where possible, to explain and help the patient to plan his own administrations at least a day or two before discharge. Written instructions do serve as useful reminders.

Patient education about drugs, their purposes and possible side effects should be planned in each health care situation. Nurses should be able to plan this in their total patient care in hospital or at home. Of course, to achieve this they need accurate, up-to-date knowledge about current drugs.

A summary of factors thought to encourage adherence is provided in Table 8.

PLACEBO EFFECTS OF MEDICATIONS

The derivation of the term 'placebo' is from the phrase 'I will please'. It is used in medicine to mean the symptom-relieving effect of some pharmacologically inert preparation or event. Historically it was customary to give certain placebo preparations which were known sometimes to relieve symptoms.

Harvard and Pearson (1977) state that on average one third of patients with symptoms such as pain or cough will respond to placebo medications and an even higher proportion of patients with psychological symptoms such as anxiety or insomnia are relieved.

The effects of giving 'sugar pills' instead of active substances have been studied to assess how positive psychological appraisal of the process of being prescribed some pills actually works. Presumably, as Rachman and Philips (1975) say, taking medicine fulfills a variety of needs which are social and psychological rather than pharmacological. In a study with neurotic patients Brill and Koegler (1964) showed that those on placebo medications improved to the same degree as others on different types of tranquillisers. Even when patients were told that they were to be prescribed some 'sugar pills' which might help them, Park and Covi (1965) found that there was a 41 per cent decrease in their symptoms. Despite the fact that they knew the pill was inert, four patients said it was the most effective pill they had taken and three patients complained of side effects.

Apparently the size and colour of pills affects their potency as placebo agents. Harvard and Pearson (1977) say: 'Blue capsules produce more sedative effects than pink capsules. Anxiety responds better to green than to red or yellow tablets. Two capsules produce more pronounced effects than one, even though the dose is the same; and the sedative and other side effects of a placebo are increased by doubling the dose'.

The major variable affecting placebo power is the behaviour of the prescribing doctor. Joyce (1962) found that patients were more likely to improve on a placebo medication when doctors expressed their faith in the pills than in those cases where they were noncommittal. Rachman and Philips (1975) also suggest that when patients respect the doctor's judgement and are aware of his personal interest in them, they are more likely to believe in his prescriptions.

There is some controversy over whether personality characteristics predisposing towards placebo reactions can be identified. Rachman and Philips claim that patients who are sociable, conventional, dependent and anxious are more likely to respond whereas those who are mistrustful and isolated tend not to respond in this way. On the other hand, research findings suggest that personality factors cannot be used as predictors of placebo response, to date. However, Shapiro, Streuning, Barten and Shapiro (1975) suggested that more research should be done with the Minnesota Multiphasic Personality Inventory (MMPI) to isolate relevant factors.

Generally, whenever a medication is prescribed some placebo effect may be expected and doctors throughout the ages have recognised this. It is now rare for a prescription for an inert substance to be given but there are exceptional occasions when this may occur. For instance if a patient visits a doctor expecting a prescription and will be dissatisfied without one, but the physician considers this to be unnecessary, he may resort to prescribing 'Vitamin C'. Likewise if all known available preparations have been tried for a chronic or terminal illness the doctor may give a placebo prescription in the hope that 'something is better than nothing'.

In order to distinguish pharmacodynamic effects of a drug from the non-pharmacological effects (i.e., placebo) an inert substance is often used in research. Direct comparisons are made on subjects given active agents with those who are given the placebo. However, as the placebo reaction itself is often quite substantial this poses great problems in interpretation. Unless the positive effects of the new drug on trial are significantly higher than those of the placebo, it cannot be said to be more therapeutic.

Because of the symptom reducing effects of doctors' communications regarding the medications, it is necessary that both the doctor and patient be unaware of the nature of the prescription during a drug trial. This situation is termed a 'double blind' trial. (A less adequate design is sometimes employed when only one person is unaware of the prescription and it is therefore called a 'single blind' trial.) The trials require the use of a placebo identical in all respects, colour, shape, weight and side effects, so that neither patient or doctor can differentiate. Because patients' intrinsic responses are so varied an alternative research strategy is to use patients 'as their own controls', that is, to give them active agents for a set period and note the effects, to then change this to the placebo and note any alteration in effects and perhaps once more return to the active drug on trial. This controls for so-called 'intrinsic patient variables' and reduces the number of people involved.

CONCLUSION

The taking of drugs and the effects they have are related to many patient and staff factors. As has been shown in this Chapter, staff can increase adherence among their patients by friendly and informative communications with them. In that part of the healing process comes from the patient's satisfaction and belief in staff, the latter should not rely on prescriptions alone for treatment. The placebo effect is clearly important and is itself therapeutic. It is therefore up to staff to help patients understand the importance of their treatments and to show their interest in them by giving a little extra reassurance.

9

Discharge from hospital and illness in the community

Leaving hospital is usually seen as a very pleasant event by most patients. However, for some it may be quite stressful. Few studies have assessed patients' reactions to discharge, possibly because so many patients are discharged at short notice, providing little time for them to plan for or adjust to the idea but also resulting in reduced opportunity for researchers to interview them. However, findings from the longitudinal study (Wilson-Barnett and Carrigy, 1978) with those in general medical wards showed that patients were not always so pleased to be discharged from hospital. (This was not only related to those who lived alone and simply appreciated being looked after by nursing staff.) From the study design of attaining a daily mood score one would anticipate anxiety and depression to be significantly less on the day of discharge in comparison with the average scores for the duration of hospitalisation. In this study one hospital sample did score significantly less depression and anxiety, as expected, but in the other hospital this was not found. Several patients were dejected for a variety of reasons. Often elderly patients were worried about the journey arrangements, of not being looked after on the train, etc., and about coping at home without very much assistance. Another small group of patients in this hospital were overtly dissatisfied at being discharged. They were either discontented with the arrangements for this, which were inadequate, or the short notice they were given but also they were unhappy to have been hospitalised for tests or consultations which did little for their condition. From these and other findings, preparations from staff would appear necessary to prevent this type of reaction.

In contrast to the dearth of studies on how patients feel about their discharge, there are several surveys of patients' experiences after discharge. Research in the community is directed towards assessing the extent of incapacity in the community, describing how hospital staff communicate with those in the community service and measuring individual patient's needs in relation to available services. These will be discussed in more detail.

THE PREVALENCE STUDIES OF ILLNESS

The first type of study, the prevalence study, is usually undertaken on a wide survey scale. Obtaining representative and reliable data about the proportions of disabled in the community is obviously necessary before administrative decisions for planning services can be made. Bennett, Garrod and Halil (1970) aimed to estimate the levels of the chronically ill and disabled in the catchment area of St. Thomas' hospital. They assessed disablement as the deficits in mobility, self-care and ability to dress and wash, to do domestic duties and to earn a living. In a two-stage survey in this area they found that 7.2 per cent of men and 9.7 per cent of women were disabled in at least one of these aspects. Rates of disability increased with age and over 75 years 34.4 per cent of men and 41.7 per cent of women fell into this category. The major causes for this disability are shown below:

Table 9 Percentage of primary diagnoses associated with disability (from Bennett, A. E., Garrod, J. and Halil, T. (1970) Chronic disease and disability in the community: a prevalence study. *British Medical Journal*, 3, 762–4; with kind permission of the editor and authors)

	Locomotor			*Internal*
	Cerebrovascular	Arthritic	Respiratory	Cardiovascular
Males	0.6	0.8	2.3	0.8
Females	0.4	1.7	1.1	0.9

The prevalence of chronic illness in the community, with particular reference to those patients discharged from hospital, had also been studied by Ferguson (1961). He studied 705 male patients discharged from acute medical wards over a two-year period from the time of their discharge. In this work the author noted that for many patients a hospital stay (even in an acute medical ward) is one stage in a chronic illness. Of this sample 18 per cent were over 64 years, 26 per cent died within the two years, 22 per cent were readmitted and only 40 per cent were likely to go back to work again in three weeks from discharge. Return to work is usually used as an indicator of complete recovery and Ferguson noted that it was more often those in skilled work that returned to full employment and doctors considered 20 per cent of this sample were actually returning to unsuitable jobs, or working below their prior capacity.

Readmission and causes for relapse were also discussed by Ferguson. 10 per cent of these readmissions could have been prevented by better health habits such as correct use of diets and drugs and 15 per cent were readmitted due to poor social and living standards and employment difficulties. Despite medical advice it was estimated that only a third of patients would adhere to medications and instructions.

Ferguson concludes that many of these problems could be reduced by more integration of services in the hospital and community and more rehabilitation centres to bridge the gap to prevent the rapid decline inevitable in bad housing and social situations.

The problems of the aged are even more severe. Brocklehurst and Shergold (1968) found 26 per cent of 200 geriatric patients followed up over two years had to be readmitted. The demands on supportive services in the community were greatest during the first month after discharge even though the majority of patients had a chronic disabling disease. Despite the already relatively heavy use of the services this study showed that 45 per cent of these patients could do with more help.

29 per cent of this sample lived with friends or relatives other than their children and some obtained places in residential homes, 30 per cent went to live with their daughter or son and it was in this group that mental stress, depression and loneliness occurred most often. Although 33 per cent of the total sample suffered substantial mental stress half of those living with their children reported this. Case studies summarised in this paper demonstrate the extreme social isolation and even cruelty which old people have to tolerate. They related how one old woman was forced to live in an upstairs room while her son and daughter-in-law occupied the remainder of the house. Her extreme isolation was highlighted by the ritual at meal times when her food was actually left outside her room by her daughter-in-law. She rarely had the opportunity to talk to anyone at all. Another instance of this appalling loneliness is cited:

Mr. B (aged 83) admitted with pneumonia lives with his son and daughter-in-law. Shunned by his daughter-in-law and barely tolerated by his son, he feels an outcast within his family circle. He seems lost and alone – 'his undisguised pleasure at seeing me, although a complete stranger, was as pathetic as it was understandable'. He is a prisoner in solitary confinement in a back bedroom lacking any touch of homeliness or comfort. He has neither radio nor books. His son rarely, his daughter-in-law never, talks to him.

MEASURING PATIENTS' NEED FOR HELP

Assessing the extent of the need for increased services in terms of staff numbers is obviously necessary but devising tools to measure individual's incapacities and requirements is perhaps more necessary for nurses. Roberts (1975) attempted to do this with a sample of 164 patients discharged from hospital. She constructed an incapacity scale and a residual incapacity scale which was a summation of all the unmet needs for care to reach a tolerable amount of independence. In effect this measured the patients' perception of their needs and the degree to which they considered these to be fulfilled. The methodology of this study was therefore useful both for research and as a continual assessment of services. Roberts pointed out that the early discharge policy of many hospitals substantially increased the load on community services. However, in this study 82 per cent said their care was altogether satisfactory despite the fact that the majority of ward sisters interviewed by Roberts put 'the discharge procedure' very low on their list of priorities.

The actual percentage of patients' comments which are unfavourable on discharge procedures and community facilities available varies between studies, but the fact that recent work in this area does reveal hardship is obviously justification enough for more effort by health workers. Skeet (1970) had three major aims for her large study in this area. They were as follows:

1. To assess what discharged patients see as their home care needs.
2. To assess how these needs are being met.
3. To describe the hospital arrangements and existing community services for discharged hospital patients.

In this study 533 patients from six general hospitals were interviewed both during their hospital stay and fourteen days after discharge.

Patients' needs at home were said to be neglected in 45 per cent of these cases. 30 per cent said they had felt 'run down' since their discharge and 16 per cent of those taking medications were worried about drugs or their side-effects. Since discharge, 28 per cent said they were unable to get sufficient pain relief because they could not obtain strong enough 'pain killers'.

The preparation for discharge given by hospital staff was found inadequate. There was little planning and 37 per cent of the patients had 24 hours or even less warning of their discharge. The surgical patients tended to get less warning than medical patients. 19 per cent of all those who were discharged needed practical assistance and 26 per cent needed information and advice and did not receive either. In all 59 per cent of these patients received no other advice than 'don't do too much' or 'take care of yourself'. To summarise, Skeet found that the majority of patients did not have any communication about their discharge and post-discharge needs.

A similar study in Scotland by Clarke (1972) also found that it was the communication which was insufficient. For instance, 25 per cent of the 376 patients in this study said they were not told what was wrong with them and 28.8 per cent said they did not receive enough information while in hospital. A fifth of these patients were told of their discharge on the same day they were discharged. 72 per cent were not asked if they needed help at home despite the fact that half of these patients admitted to being less active than before their stay in hospital. GPs in this study were also dissatisfied with communications from the hospital, a fifth regretted the delay in full summaries from the hospital medical staff. They commented, in particular, that they were rarely told of the patients transfer to another hospital or of their death.

LIVING WITH A CHRONIC ILLNESS

If one considers that hospitalisation is just one stage in chronic illness, the care of chronically ill patients in community and in hospital should necessitate close links between the two services. The care after discharge from hospital may well prevent further admissions and the amount of information a community physician or nurse receives from the hospital may well influence how efficiently this care is given. In addition, if emotional stress results in a reduced capacity to cope with illness both physically and psychologically, it is even more vital to give care and support which might prevent this.

Patients' experiences in the community may well be frustrating and fragmentation of services may increase this. Strauss (1975) has studied how patients live with chronic illness and the sort of problems they experience. Although this is an American sociological study the depth of information offers great insight.

Strauss pointed out that about half the USA population suffers from some chronic disorder and reiterated that most patients in hospital are not there for treatment of an acute illness but for assessment or care during an exacerbation of their condition. He listed the main elements of living with a condition that require adaptation as:

1. Prevention and management of medical crises.
2. Control of symptoms.
3. Carrying out prescribed regimens.
4. Prevention of or living with social isolation.
5. Adjustment to fluctuations in the course of the disease.
6. Attempts at normalising behaviour.
7. Financing treatment in the face of unemployment.

Many aspects of a patient's life were discussed by Strauss. For instance, adherence to regimens obviously may affect individual activities which have to be rearranged around a strict time schedule. The family and friends may then also be affected by this routine. Being obliged to adjust, they may not always be co-operative. Coping with various symptoms may be even more disruptive. In colitis, for example, frequent trips to the toilet may curb social outings and restrict the type of occupation which is possible. New strategies for doing even the most ordinary things often have to be employed. Patients with a heart condition which leaves them very weak may become very skilful in slipping behind someone as they cannot open the door themselves. Patients become very resourceful and many clever tactics are employed for coping.

Planning is, or course, dependent on knowing the type and expected severity of symptoms. 'Surprises' are the hardest to cope with and therefore most debilitating. Sudden incontinence or weakness is both distressing and damaging to patients' attempts at being independent and active. If they occur too frequently, invalidism may result prematurely.

Relationships with family and friends are often very strained when they all realise that a chronic disease is going to be a permanent feature of the patient's and their own life. Strauss says it is like living with a different person who has different abilities, habits and roles. The reaction of others may be to isolate further the sick person. Thus social isolation can be just as real for those who live with their family as for those who cope on their own. Attempts to normalise or pretend that nothing is wrong often lead to long-term difficulties. If the patient manages to do something one day and then fails on the next the family may consider that they are not trying so hard. Those with a condition with spontaneous remissions such as multiple sclerosis find it very hard to explain to others that they are not in control of how much they can or cannot do.

Attempts to 'normalise' while experiencing pain may also lead to long-term misfortune. The strain for a rheumatic who tries to walk straight while in pain, in order not to attract attention or embarrass others, may in fact cause much worse pain for a long time afterwards. Strauss tells of the patient who could only manage to walk if she walked backwards. This was obviously very inconvenient, but it was mainly other people's reactions which prevented her outings. He also mentioned the case of a man who was so used to pain that he did not realise he had a broken leg for a month.

This type of social constraint is seen with many chronic illnesses. Both the patient and their family often go through many coping strategies either eventually to succeed or if they are inadequate the patient's condition may deteriorate beyond the resources of self and family help. In which case social agencies have to be employed and hospitalisation may be recurrent.

How well do the services available in the United Kingdom realise the needs in the community, and are there sufficient resources to cope with the growing demands in the community? Already areas of neglect have been identified by the studies mentioned above but a rather different orientation to this question was employed by Hockey (1968), who asked, 'whether district services to discharged in-patients and out-patients could be increased?'. After interviewing over 3000 patients from six hospitals she concluded that the majority of simple nursing and household tasks were being shouldered by the patient or family, the contribution of the home help service being negligible in relation to the substantial need. Athough most major nursing needs were met, patients had many unresolved anxieties and problems.

GPs thought the existing district nursing services were inadequate and that attachment schemes for nurses with general practice units was advisable. Once more communications between the hospital and district nursing services was on the whole sparse and paucity of information about patients was mutually regretted. However, although ward sisters and district nurses seemed to complain about this, they did little to relieve the problem.

19 per cent of these patients had need of something at home, the type of needs whereas outlined in Table 10.

Table 10

Patients' needs at home	%
Domestic or simple nursing help	33
Medical or nursing advice and reassurance	30
Other services	27
Financial help	26
Convalescence	11
Advice about housing and employment	9

Research findings of an earlier study by Hockey (1966) showed that district nurses spent 'surprisingly little time' nursing patients and that the help they gave frequently did not require their nursing expertise. They frequently lacked information to care for their patients and had little contact with hospital nurses, GPs or health visitors. Doctors were ignorant of the district nurses' abilities and qualifications and consequently under-used them, but they considered that the service could be widened to meet their patients' needs.

In an attempt to assess services for psychiatric patients, Sainsbury (1973) compared a 'new community care' (Chichester) service with a traditional service (Salisbury). Referrals to the psychiatric team in the Chichester area rose sharply after the extra staff and facilities were introduced. These included more community social workers, nursing homes and more consultant domiciliary visits. The admissions to hospital were halved during the two years of this study and it was usually found to be social factors which finally influenced admissions. Sainsbury concluded that 'the community care policy was preferentially providing a service for the seriously mentally disordered in the community who had previously been neglected'.

However, comparisons between areas for the burden placed on families of patients showed that 'community care' meant a much higher burden. Further investigation was said to show this was only true for those families without adequate social support, i.e., 'the combined skills of a therapeutic team and GP'.

In conclusion it seems that these findings point to certain recommendations. An awareness of the need by personnel is surely the first necessity to improve services. Health visitors, district nurses and social workers can all have a vital function in detecting needs but also in providing a co-ordinated service. Skeet's recommendations (1970) are still relevant, and the major ones, summarised below, serve to illustrate the deficiencies suffered by many patients:

1. Two-way communication between hospital and community regarding home and domestic arrangements.
2. Adequate notice of discharge dates.
3. Written instructions on diets and drugs, etc.
4. Adequate clerical staff to enable discharge communications to be sent.
5. Planned after-care organised with GP and community services.
6. Routine counselling from health visitors for recently discharged patients.
7. Sufficient district nurses and social workers for assessing and giving services.
8. Adequate supervision of facilities.
9. Care in half-way houses.
10. Door to door transport services.
11. Home help and meals-on-wheels operating daily.
12. Night sitter services.
13. Voluntary helpers for cooking, gardening, shopping and laundry.
14. Voluntary relief services for relatives.
15. More information and publicity about available help.

10

Reactions to malignant disease and to death and bereavement

This section aims to trace emotional reactions of the patients, their families and those who care for them to the development of malignant conditions. As Maguire (1978) says, cancer may be seen as a most psychologically disturbing event likened to a stressful life event with major loss. All the emotional responses, he suggests, are greater and more intense than for any other disease.

Emotional reactions are thought to vary according to personality factors, to meaning attributed to 'cancer', to the experience of hospitalisation and to social roles and aspirations. All these factors also influence a persons behaviour and may affect prognosis throughout the course of a malignant disease. Patients' relationships with their family and the staff and their expression of both their awareness and emotions will also interrelate in a complex and often changeable way.

The progression of cancer has been traditionally divided into stages as outlined by Abrams (1974):

Stage I: The localised or primary stage which has a good prognosis.
Stage II: With regional involvement when there is spread from the primary site. This may be controllable, the prognosis is therefore 'fair' to 'guarded'.
Stage III: The advanced stage with metastases, where the prognosis is 'guarded' to 'poor' and care is directed to provide physical and emotional comfort.

In this section it is planned to discuss reactions, problems of communication and care and the ideal goals of care with reference to each stage, from diagnosis to death. In many of these aspects there is a paucity of systematic information but much 'informed' opinion. This review is anything but comprehensive but may provide starting points for further reading in a subject where doctors and nurses have much to learn and contribute.

THE DIAGNOSTIC PROCESS

It is a puzzling fact that at least two studies have found that patients who are actually suffering from cancer tend to also be more anxious and depressed even before they are diagnosed. Maguire (1978) studied women with lumps in their breast, who were unaware of their diagnosis at the time of biopsy and found those with malignant lumps were more anxious and depressed than those with benign lumps. They explained that this was due to the thought that it might be cancer rather than they might have to lose their breast. Wilson-Barnett (1977) also found that those (as yet undiagnosed patients) who were found to have cancer were more anxious than others at the time of a diagnostic X-ray. As mentioned previously, in the medical ward sample studied by the author (Wilson-Barnett, 1978) the 'malignant disease' group of patients also reported more feelings of anxiety and depression throughout their hospital stay than others. These emotions may be due to certain clues which physicians may unwittingly have given but general tiredness and depression has been suggested a prodromal indication of a malignant disorder (see Ch. 2).

At this diagnostic stage Abrams (1974) says conversation and communications are quite open. Although it is a stressful time, doctors are able to be optimistic about outcome and the patient can talk freely to their family and doctor. In contrast, Maguire's (1978) study compared patients (100) with malignant lumps with those who had benign lumps (80) and found that from the total sample 73 per cent were worried and 85 per cent were aware it could be cancer but felt unable to communicate fully with staff about their fears.

Smith (1976) considers that reactions to a diagnosis of cancer may be more severe to one who has responsibilities and an earning capacity, but makes certain assumptions about implications which may not be shared by the patient. She assumes that:

1. Most patients want to know if they have cancer.
2. All patients with malignant disease have some awareness of it.
3. The majority of patients understand something about their treatment and know it is associated with malignant disease.

She outlines a scheme of emotional reactions to cancer:

1. A stunned reaction.
2. Hopelessness, anxiety, hostility.
3. Guilt, self-blame.
4. Repression or denial and projection of blame.
5. Disruption of adaptive patterns and major reorganisation.

6. Ongoing anxiety and uncertainty.
7. Conscious avoidance.
8. Preoccupation with the disease.
9. Complaints and excessive demands for nursing attention.
10. Fear of speaking openly about cancer.

At this early stage, admission to a hospital for tests may cause more immediate emotional reactions than the reason for the tests. Perhaps the patient's experiences are exemplified in this passage from Thompson (1978), the Chaplain at the Royal Marsden Hospital: 'He leaves behind a full diary and enters a world in which he sits around waiting for things to happen. All his most personal functions are monitored and of public interest. He is often spoken to as though he had no intelligence, and as though his disease were part of the property of the hospital rather than part of himself. He presents his tumour to the hospital and hands over all responsibility for it.'

This is far from an ideal situation as Thompson considers everyone should be in control of their destiny and should know about their own investigations and be able to express their feelings.

SURGICAL INTERVENTION FOR TREATMENT OF CANCER

The consequences of surgery for primary cancer have been discussed by Maguire (1975 and 1978). Not only do they lead to much psychological morbidity but they seem to cause difficulties for staff to act in an empathic and communicative way. This situation seems to be more marked than for other types of surgery. Once surgery has been deemed necessary, patients are more likely to realise that the 'tumour' or 'ulcer' or 'growth' was extensive. Their realisation, or likelihood of realising, the severity or even malignant nature of their illness becomes part of their stress post-operatively.

Maguire's studies have concentrated on mastectomy patients. His findings point to the severity and long lasting nature of psychological distress of these patients. Both the fear of cancer spreading and leading to their death and the grieving over the loss of a breast caused moderate or marked depression in 32 per cent of these patients in the three-month period after operation, while 83 per cent suffered from depression in the full year following operation. The relationships both with their husbands and with friends deteriorated because of their low morale and feelings of worthlessness due to their 'unattractive' and 'scarred' body. 46 per cent of those who previously had a regular and satisfying sex life reported a definite decline in sexual relations. Many of them would no longer sleep in the same bed as their husband and 13 per cent concealed the scar from their husband. Their life became very hard for them and they even had difficulty coping with their routine housework.

If radiotherapy was necessary for these patients they often saw this as a sign of spread or that the operation had not been successful. It was, therefore, associated with an increase in the amount of anxiety, depression and fatigue which peaked six weeks after radiotherapy was completed.

Another operation which affects physical appearance and engenders feelings of 'being different' or even a 'freak' was studied by Devlin, Plant and Griffin (1971). Their research with patients who had ano-rectal surgery and formation of permanent colostomies showed similar features to Maguire's work. They compared 83 of these patients with 38 who had restorative surgery after a temporary colostomy. 23 per cent of the former group had had psychiatric problems, mainly of depression and sometimes with obsessional ritualism, particularly in relation to their bowel habits and colostomy care. The main concerns were those of insecurity over when they would have an 'action' and of the 'odour'. Because of these fears 35 per cent of these patients had reduced their social contacts with others. Many of those over 64 had a problem of isolation which was five times greater than for the normal population. Their personal relationships were also affected. Many had a fear of sex, partly because of fear of spillage but also because of a realistic fear of impotence due to the likelihood of nerves to the erector muscles having been severed. This usually led to friction in the marriage.

The great problem of hidden psychological morbidity, Maguire (1978) considers, is mainly due to the staff's lack of enquiry into how their patients are adjusting to their illness and treatment. Most of the staff's work is focused on physical well-being. The problem of lack of this communication about patients' needs was studied by Maguire (1976). He monitored staff's interaction with patients in hospital and recorded their conversations. Mention of mood or feelings by staff was extremely rare. Another study by Maguire (1978) found that surgeons actually professed to say certain things to their patients, yet, when observed, this was patently not so, as patients' desire for information or attention to their anxiety reactions was never really tackled by these doctors. In this study the researchers found that 17 per cent of these patients were actually told they did not have cancer and were, therefore, very distrustful when they returned from theatre after a mastectomy.

Maguire (1978) points out that there is really inadequate evidence on whether patients should be told they have cancer and their prognosis when it is either regionally or generally spread. What usually happens is probably very unsatisfactory as Abrams (1974) describes this stage when communication becomes disruptive, cautious and evasive. The patient may be presented to more and more doctors and is told less and less about what is happening. As she says, 'paradoxically the patient becomes less open but more dependent on the physician as the disease progresses. Haunted by a nagging fear of rejection, he becomes uncomplaining, good, passive, overly nice and overly co-operative'.

Glaser and Strauss (1965) discuss four main types of communication between staff and patients which flow in such situations. These are:

1. *Closed awareness*. The patient does not know of impending death although everyone else does. Most patients do not know how to recognise signs of a fatal disease and doctors rationalise that if they want to know their prognosis they will find out anyway. Their families tend to guard the secret although this leads to a stressful non-disclosure drama. Nurses, too, find guarding against disclosure difficult and are often very relieved when this becomes unnecessary.

2. *Suspected awareness*. The patient may suspect that everyone else knows their prognosis. Staff's reactions are as for (1).

3. *Mutual pretence awareness*. Both patient and staff know about the prognosis but pretend they do not. They follow implicit rules where both avoid dangerous areas of conversation and daily routines and symptoms become the focus of conversation. This pretence may preclude a close relationship with the patient and his family because of the strain of interaction.

4. *Awareness*. Although this makes communication less strained, the patient becomes responsible for his actions and is expected to act in a dignified way.

Research to find whether patients wish to be told about their diagnosis and prognosis is usually retrospective. McIntosh's (1976) study of cancer patients was said to show that it is unnecessary for patients to be told their diagnosis. 74 patients with diagnosed but undisclosed malignancy were interviewed to ascertain their awareness and desire for information. 88 per cent knew or suspected they had a tumour but apparently the great majority had no wish to augment that knowledge. The conclusion to this study was: 'The fact that their diagnosis or prognosis was not revealed to them allowed many patients to maintain the hope that either they might not have cancer or that the outlook might be favourable'.

McIntosh considered that there was no need to give explicit information to patients as they will always be able to find out for themselves. The treatment they receive will be a clear clue, the fact that they were not told of their diagnosis is confirmation that it is cancer and they can usually make deductions from seeing other patients and what is actually said to them by the doctor. All this, he says, is sufficiently ambiguous to maintain hope.

Another survey of 219 doctors cited by Lipowski (1975) showed how typical McIntosh's views are, as 90 per cent said they did not usually disclose the diagnosis of cancer.

Unfortunately if patients are fearful and not given clear explanation of their condition and treatment their fantasies may be even more terrifying than the reality. Aitken-Swan and Easson (1959) obtained very different responses from their patients. Of 231 patients told of their diagnosis of cancer, only 7 per cent said they would rather not have been told, while the great majority wished to know their diagnosis. All these patients had a curable form of cancer, yet 19 per cent of them later denied that they had been told of their diagnosis. Oken (1961) also found that 87 per cent of 630 patients wanted to know their diagnosis of cancer.

This dichotomy of view over whether patients should be told their diagnosis really makes it more of a moral debate rather than a therapeutic one. Should perhaps just certain patients be told of their diagnosis, and do doctors have sufficient wisdom to judge which of their patients should be told? Brewin (1977) discussed this issue and advised that doctors should take time to assess each patient's ability to adjust to cancer and a poor prognosis. Despite this he also gives more reasons why doctors should be very cautious in giving information. As he says, 'even the patient himself is sometimes not sure exactly what he fears, or what he already knows, or suspects, or wants to know, about the seriousness of his condition'.

He suggests that one may learn more about the patient's need from their second question rather than the first. Some can tolerate a poor prognosis rather than the fact they have cancer, others are the exact opposite. He considers that those who are told and then deny their illness should not really have been told and furthermore should not be threatened by direct questions about their feelings.

Whatever communications occur it is therefore important to be sensitive to patient cues, to listen in order to assess whether they require more knowledge and to create an easy atmosphere for them to express their views. Maguire (1978) states that on the rare occasions where counselling occurs before and after operation for cancer of the breast, psychological distress is much reduced. It is, perhaps, only right to give patients the chance to adjust and accept their illness which has a guarded prognosis rather than suppressing information, often, it seems, because staff are ill-prepared to counsel patients or are too anxious themselves to be able to face patients' distress. As Thompson (1978) says, those staff who claim patients do not want to know their diagnosis are often missing their patients' hints and subtle invitations to discuss this subject. The fewer communications there are, he surmises, the less confidence the patient will have and the less chance for co-operating in his treatment.

Nurses are also apparently inadequate at comforting or communicating with distressed patients who have cancer. In the breast clinic Maguire (1975) noted that nurses did not pick up verbal or non-verbal cues which were given by patients. Even if women were crying or weeping staff never enquired of them the reasons for this and therefore never gave them any reassurance. The consequence of this was that women rarely took the opportunity to talk about their condition as they didn't want to seem silly and felt it was inappropriate to express their worries to people who were primarily concerned with patients' physical health. They usually left the clinic in a very worried state. This research showed that there was generally inadequate opportunity to ask questions or discuss their worries and even when a consent form had to be signed the possibility of mastectomy was glossed over or denied and always without opportunity for discussion with their husbands before agreeing. In summary, Maguire says: 'Many of the surgical and nursing staff seemed reluctant to talk to these women about their feelings. They found it easier to give sedation and offer ineffective reassurances'.

Treatment during times of localised and regionally involved cancer should be aimed at physical and psychological adjustment. Maguire (1978) outlines aims for such rehabilitation as follows:

1. To achieve as full a physical recovery as possible.
2. To come to terms with any residual physical disabilities of mutilation.
3. To learn to live with the possibility of recurrence.
4. To return to their previous way of life.

Implicit in these aims is a strong, understanding relationship between staff and patients. Three of these aims require a supportive role for the nurse or other staff member to help the patient think through the coping strategies implied. To do this staff must have the inclination to interact, to listen and to empathise.

THE ADVANCED STAGE

In the advanced stage of cancer there may be many aspects of care which relieve symptoms, such as nerve blocks, palliative operations and drugs or radio therapy. At this stage in illness it is not usual to call a patient terminal. This only occurs when no further active treatment is undertaken and when the life expectancy is in terms of months or weeks.

As the disease progresses, most patients get more and more dependent on their doctors and nurses, which often makes their family feel helpless and unneeded. Patients may initially wonder whether a change of doctor may help, even at this stage, and often attempt to find a cause for their condition in terms of their own or someone else's fault (Abrams, 1974). But at this time Lipowski (1975) notes that the doctor, in an attempt to cope with his own sense of failure, becomes awkward and detached. This only serves to increase the patient's sense of helplessness and loneliness.

At this stage the family will also need support and advice. Abrams (1974) says that if the patient is able to communicate about his condition his family may find it easier to be close. If they cry at the bedside this is a clear indication to the patient that he is loved. This may strangely give him strength at this lonely time. The family should be told that the patient's reactions of denial or awareness may alternate and they should try to satisfy his needs at all times without forcing him to be acceptant when he does not have the strength. As Smith (1976) says, when the patient is physically more fit he may be able to accept and adjust more easily. Hardest of all for everyone to bear are the silences which patients require.

If denial or regression are prevalent Abrams considers that it is up to the care-giver to decide whether or not these hamper communication and a worthwhile acceptance of reality or palliative treatment and should be corrected. They may, of course, enable the patient to maintain a tolerable life which otherwise would be impossible despite the strain it puts on the family.

During this stage Abrams (1974) says that reactions alternate between surges of hope and despondency, between tremendous efforts at independence and the need to lean on others. Nurses should learn to adapt to these different needs and comply supportively.

CARE OF THE TERMINALLY ILL

At the terminal stage of any illness patients often have no strength to do things for themselves and become emotionally detached or calmly suspended in hopelessness (Abrams, 1974). Silence, she says, is most needed at this time, while empathy and support for reactions should be shown. Although nursing is difficult to carry out in the home, frequently the family request this. Many philosophers, social scientists and therapists claim that isolation is the main factor which causes distress at this stage. In familiar surroundings this is less likely to occur.

Summers (1978) provides guidance for health workers to help the patient in becoming close to his family and achieving some individual goal which gives him satisfaction. Such opportunities, she says, are of great importance to the patient.

An alternative approach to treatment is provided by Yalom and Greaves (1977) who advise active psychological group therapy for the terminally ill. They undertook a four-year group study with patients who had metastatic cancer who attended 90-minute sessions aimed at moving them out of self-absorption to being helped by helping others. Altruism, catharsis, group cohesiveness and existential factors were the main mechanisms for this help. The researchers noted that a great amount of anger was expressed by these patients at their desertion by medical staff at the terminal stage of illness. Their anxieties were not so related to dying or non-being but to loneliness and isolation, which was said to be prevented by the existence of the group.

Many of these points are reiterated by Weisman (1975) in his psychiatric liason work. He points out that the psychiatrist is usually called in when a patient is becoming a behaviour problem or a disturbance. The problems are usually related to fears of abandonment at time of physical deterioration and annihilation. Depression, of course, is part of expecting nothing of oneself in the future and this becomes the dying person's outlook. Disappointments and frustrations, uncertainty and disillusionment have occurred and still occur for someone who is terminally ill. The psychological sufferings are said to mainly arise due to vulnerability at the hands of others. Feelings of alienation, endangerment, encroachment and destruction usually lead to periods of intense dysphoria.

These terminal patients must be restored to a rightfully safe position, says Weisman where their significance is endorsed by sufficient communication, compassion, concern and intelligent use of support systems.

The strain of nursing at home, Glaser and Strauss (1975) consider may well be worth it in terms of the patient's experience. At home the patient does not have to compete for attention with other patients and does not have to be seen by other patients. They note that American nurses also may deny the patient opportunity to talk about death and this usually leads to mutual pretence. Because the nurses find it difficult to talk about dying, most patients are sensitive enough to remain silent. However, Cartwright, Hockey and Anderson's (1973) study revealed many of the problems which occur when terminally ill patients are cared for at home. District nurses were 'too rushed' to talk to patients and there was a great need for more help in the home. Patients often had very distressing symptoms which had not been communicated to their doctor. A large proportion of patients in the year before their death suffered from pain, sleeplessness, loss of bladder and bowel control and vomiting. All these were nursing and domestic problems which usually put a great strain on the relatives. In addition, the relatives were frequently harrassed by poor communications between health workers.

DEATH AND DYING

Kubler Ross (1969) from her famous study of interviews and seminars with dying patients notes that 'if a patient is allowed to terminate his life in the familiar and beloved environment it requires less adjustment for him'. By making death impersonal, mechanical and isolated, staff are the ones who are protected from distress, not the patient. From talking, in depth, to over 200 patients a pattern of reactions to dying were found. These stages are not necessarily discrete or ordered and they may last for different lengths of time for each individual. They are:

1. *Denial.* Although short lived, most patients react by saying 'No – not me'.
2. *Anger.* This is often projected at staff or even the family.
3. *Bargaining.* In an attempt to win a reprieve, many seek to offer certain services to medical staff.
4. *Depression.* A typical reaction to any loss in life. It may be a necessary stage before adjustment.
5. *Acceptance.* Although this may be the goal, it is often almost void of feelings. Tiredness may prevent conversation but patients should not be forgotten. Visitors should be faithful even if they just sit quietly.
6. *Hope.* Hope exists for all during all the other stages.

The ultimate goal of acceptance is seen by Kubler Ross, Glaser and Strauss and many others as beneficial for the patient, his relatives and for the staff. It leads to more open communication and more meaningful support. It also prevents the reaction of embarrassment observed by Glaser and Strauss which caused nurses to spend less time with the patient or to direct their attention only to his physical needs.

Certain responses to the awareness that death is imminent or that 'nothing more can be done' make acceptance more difficult. Reactions of sustained denial, anger or depression may complicate acceptance and prevent a more peaceful and comfortable end. Kubler Ross talks of denial and mentions how this may be used at certain times, on certain days, by patients who may have previously accepted and talked about dying. Nurses may find this difficult to adjust to but knowledge that it is necessary for the patient's psychological integrity may help them to 'tune in' to these needs. Anger or hostility reactions may also lead to isolation of the patient and difficulty in learning to talk through his fears. Hostility is usually related to fears of death and may be reduced if nurses and relatives discuss the patients feelings with patience and kindness.

Perhaps the most serious reaction to knowledge of imminent death is that of guilt. As Kubler Ross says, this is 'the most painful companion of death'. A psychiatrist may be needed to help in exploring the patient's feelings and methods for resolving this reaction. Reassurance from relatives is sometimes very comforting for such patients.

Many more problematic reactions are due to a block in communications and a trusting relationship between staff and patients at the time when they accept that the patient is near death. Staff are often so distressed by their inability to help patients further that they cannot bring themselves to talk about future plans for care. Patients frequently learn from various cues that their symptoms are to be managed conservatively and that no more active investigations or treatments will occur. It seems evident from research that opportunities for patients to talk should be created and that each patient may express their needs differently, although an overall pattern of reactions may exist.

Kubler Ross concludes her account by saying: 'to summarise briefly what these patients have taught us, the outstanding fact, to my mind, is that they are all aware of the seriousness of their illness whether they are told or not. They do not always show this knowledge with their doctor or next of kin. The reason for this is that it is painful to think of such a reality and any implicit or explicit message not to talk about it is usually perceived by the patient and – for the moment – gladly accepted. There came a time, however, when all of our patients had a need to show some of their concerns, to lift the mask, to face reality, and to take care of vital matters while there was still time'.

PSYCHOLOGICAL REACTIONS TO BEREAVEMENT

Many of the patient's reactions to his own fatal illness are shared by his relatives. They, too, frequently experience initial shock and denial which gradually changes to anger and depression. Most of the advice given to staff in their support of patients is reiterated for the benefit of their relatives, as Kubler Ross says: 'let the relative talk, cry or scream if necessary. Let them share and ventilate, but be available'.

It is obviously so much more comfortable for all involved with a dying patient if staff learn how to comfort people in their time of bereavement so that grief is accepted and can be understood without embarrassment or evasion. Grief will probably be experienced when the relatives realise how seriously ill the patient is and this may become more intense as they anticipate his death. Awareness of this may come gradually through indirect cues or a direct communication. An American study by Glaser and Strauss (1965) provides great insight into the complexities and varieties of institutionalised methods of coping with bereavement adopted by relatives and staff. Their classification of knowledge of a fatal illness (see above) is applied to communications between staff, patients and their relatives. Although this may not be totally relevant to British health care, the discussion of these issues is of wide interest to all health professionals.

When the patient dies the formal bereavement period commences, however a spouse may have commenced this process during the terminal illness period. Research into the experience of bereavement has provided guidelines for supporting the bereaved. Lindeman's (1944) early work described how the recently bereaved suffered from emotional, cognitive and somatic changes. Many emotions were felt but tension and depression were most common. Guilt and anger were also experienced and these were thought to require intervention as they were often unrealistic and led to social isolation. Widows were shown 'to feel unreal', to search for their loved one continuously and be preoccupied with thoughts and images of him. They would also experience a withdrawal from social interaction, friendships lacked warmth and this led to further isolation. The physical signs included 'waves' of nausea, shortness of breath, choking and 'mental pain'. These would typically be felt when the husband was mentioned and remembered and often persisted for several years after bereavement.

Parkes (1972) also observed this syndrome and studied others who had suffered loss. He compared the reactions of the recently widowed with patients who were amputees and drew many analogies between their responses. They usually felt shock, pangs of grief and then depression and apathy. Both groups had visions of what they had lost and suffered a sense of mutilation and vulnerability. He also described those most vulnerable, particularly those who were young, left without family or those who felt ambivalent about their former marriage.

During adjustment to loss it is necessary to unlearn various habits and to learn new ways of receiving gratification and purpose for living. Glaser and Strauss, Parkes and Lindeman stress that adjustment is usually less prolonged or complicated if there is a prior awareness that loss will occur. Wives can adjust to the death of their husband if they witness his illness and 'share' his dying rather than the awful shock of sudden death with no 'rehearsal' for coping. Support and sympathy for relatives at times of hospital care for the terminally ill is the responsibility of all hospital staff caring for the patient. This is made more possible when the relatives and patient are aware of imminent death, as Glaser and Strauss emphasise but there are ways in which staff can help the wife or husband or a patient to be 'united' at the end rather than estranged by the hospital environment and procedures. For instance, staff should allow a wife the opportunity to be attentive and give care at the bedside but this should not automatically be expected. The family's wish for social activity and 'relief' from visiting should also be accepted. In other words, just as the patient's wishes for communication and support should be respected, so should those of his family.

Psychotherapy for the recently bereaved has been discussed and assessed by Glick, Weiss and Parkes (1974). Not all those who are bereaved will benefit from this specialised attention but when employed, they advise that it should be directed towards helping with the process of realising that death has occurred and to accepting that pain may continue but in the future activities will gradually seem more rewarding and purposeful. It appears from the studies mentioned that expression of grief is a beneficial means of progressing through the adjustment process.

Parkes considered that too little or too much grieving were more likely to lead to complications. He stressed that there was no ideal duration for grieving but that this should not be allowed to overwhelm everyday activities of living. Gentle encouragement for a widow to start new ventures may be helpful, but these must be realistic and not over-demanding. A part-time job may be enough to start with as further stress at an anxious, insecure time is undesirable. He also said that the frequent suggestion for people to get away 'for a while' and 'forget' only postponed adjustment and caused renewed pain on their return.

To conclude, it would, therefore, appear that community services have a potentially important role in preventing both physical and psychological illness after bereavement. The job of the staff is not over when a patient dies; both hospital and community staff must recognise the need for an expression of grief. Relatives need support at the time of and before death in order to prepare themselves for the loss, but this may also be required for a long time, months or years, afterwards. Once more, it seems that understanding, empathy and encouragement are appreciated by people who are sad and depressed.

11

Conclusion

From research discussed in the preceding Chapters it seems clear that professionals should be developing ways to prevent unnecessary distress for their patients and to help in their adjustment to illness and health care. Unfortunately there is very little research which assesses particular methods for preventing and alleviating distress, although there is a substantial body of documented advice for doctors and nurses on this subject. The advice included here is based on the writings of many authors and is reviewed in order to provide some guidelines for those helping patients. Hopefully in the future some of the advice can be examined in research studies.

RECOGNISING ANXIOUS AND DEPRESSED PATIENTS

Before discussing methods to alleviate distress, early signs of anxiety and depression are presented so that staff can intervene in an attempt to prevent major psychological problems in their patients. Aitken and Zealley's (1970) outline analysis of anxiety signs is very helpful. They mention changes in thinking, such as worry, dread and apprehension with reduced concentration and field of attention. Distractability, forgetfulness, irritability and depression are also often seen in anxiety and can be concurrent with insomnia. Motor activity disturbances include muscular tension and trembling, restlessness, fidgeting, inco-ordination and impaired performance. The somatic changes, dependent on heightened sympathetic arousal, include sweating, anorexia, tachypnoea, hyperventilation, fatigue, weakness and dyspepsia. Alteration in regularity of body functions such as defaecation and menstruation may also occur if this emotional experience persists.

It is important to observe for these changes in patients' behaviour and conversation, and unless nurses in particular are watching for these specific changes their relevance may be missed. Of course, the signs of anxiety may be masked by the patient and it may be difficult, for instance, to detect whether someone is talking more rapidly than normal or whether their conversation masks messages of fear. It therefore helps to know one's patients before they are likely to become anxious, but this is often impossible in the present pattern of rapid turnover of patients in a ward.

For the longer-term patients with chronic illness or major surgical treatment, anxiety and depression may be combined, anxiety reactions occurring in the face of many uncertainties and depressive responses in the situation of a life-threatening event of major surgery or a life-time of illness. The complex pattern of visible signs of depression, include many of those listed for anxiety but others are characteristic of depression. These include withdrawal from social interchange to become preoccupied with one's own feelings and situation, sudden bouts of tearfulness, a sad facial expression with a general lack of smiles, an outlook of pessimism, helplessness, guilt and worthlessness, sleep disturbance (particularly early morning waking) and complaints of multiple vague symptoms. There is also a general slowing of movements, retardation and loss of appetite.

When assessing if any such changes have occurred in patients, their relatives can be of great value. They obviously have greater knowledge of how the patient usually behaves and reacts to events and asking for their assessment of the patient will probably relieve their own concerns in this matter.

In general, a lack of reaction from the patient to events or aspects of treatment may indicate depression, whereas heightened over-reaction may indicate anxiety. The two emotions may be experienced as a complex and although this sometimes can be seen as a normal reaction to physical illness it does not admonish staff from an important responsibility to support and help those patients who experience them. When these reactions persist for more than a day or two, staff should decide whether to refer the patient for psychiatric help.

PREVENTING AND ALLEVIATING ANXIETY

Prevention and alleviation of anxiety in relation to 'special tests' and operations has been discussed in Chapters 5 and 6. It seems explicit that if anxiety can be redefined (Spielberger, 1972) as fear of the unknown, it can, therefore, be alleviated by explanation and fore-warning about the future. Johnson (1966) and Hayward (1975) talk about the type of information that is useful for patients prior to stressful events. They both say that it is important to inform patients about what they will feel and see. Johnson, Morrisey and Leventhal (1973) made a point of emphasising the patients' sensations during introduction of a gastroscope. They found that it helped if patients knew how this procedure would feel and how long they had to tolerate discomfort. When patients had this knowledge they could then plan how to cope with events and feel less dependent and more in control of what was happening.

Hayward also stressed that relevant information for patients was that which helped them to anticipate their experiences and prepare for them. For instance, patients who were told that they could ask for analgesia when necessary felt less fear of pain. Also, when they knew that many patients were given intravenous infusions of whole blood after operation, they were less afraid of dire surgical complications when they, too, were given blood.

It is essential when giving this information for staff to be familiar themselves with procedures and operations. It is also advisable to ask the patient if he has any initial questions before giving further explanation. This will help him to benefit from and retain more of what is being said. Patients do not usually require very technical explanations, some do have many questions to ask and staff should be able both to spare time to answer them and to give accurate information. Although explanations should prepare patients for what will definitely happen it is as well, in the case of surgery, to explain a few of the possible occurrences, such as use of drips or drains. Although it is not always possible to explain everything in advance one can reduce the unexpected to a minimum which most patients can then cope with more easily.

Staff should really be able to explain all the tests that their patients experience. If it is impossible for everyone to witness special tests or nurse patients with certain conditions, it may be feasible to get explanations from those who are familiar with them and also from patients who have had tests, to assess how they felt and what they experienced throughout. It is recommended that nurses should have time to visit specialised diagnostic departments to learn about the tests.

PLANNING FOR GIVING INFORMATION

Without some ward strategy or plan for routine explanation to patients, giving information may be sporadic and incomplete. Bird (1955) reiterated this valuable point claiming it is the systematic plan for giving information and explanation which is necessary for good pre-operative care. Each ward should assign a member of staff to provide such psychological care to particular patients so they may benefit from a continuous relationship with one special nurse or doctor. In this way a more accurate assessment of the patient's level of understanding about medical matters, illness and hospital can be made in order to give the explanation accordingly. The staff member can then also identify how anxious the patient is and whether they might benefit from discussions on how they can plan and prepare for events.

Rehearsal for positive appraisal of fearful thoughts (as described by Janis and Mann, 1976) may appear a sophisticated technique to apply in the busy surgical ward, but we already frequently suggest alternative perspectives for our patients. For instance, when they express fear of the operation, it is almost second nature to remind them of the long term advantages of less pain, etc., in the future after surgery.

Likewise, with admission to hospital it seems that patients are helped by a gradual introduction to and explanation of ward routines. It is helpful for nurses to ask the patient what he wants to know, whether he has been in hospital before, if he knows the duration of his stay, what treatment or tests are planned, and lastly whether he received a hospital booklet about routines and facilities. By asking these questions nurses at once indicate concern for the patient's feelings and gain some insight into their level of understanding. Apart from making a real attempt at empathising with a new patient the nurse should, as Robinson (1972) says, compare her efforts at hospitality and friendship in the hospital setting with those she may make when acting as a hostess in her own home.

Hospital booklets are often designed with great care but many give the impression that it is a communication for teaching hospital rules rather than helping the patient to adjust. Useful extra pieces of information include the nurses' names, when they change shifts, the best time to shower or bath (when appropriate) and how to use the mobile telephone.

EXPLANATION IN INTENSIVE CARE UNITS

In all these situations information should be given in a careful, attentive way and should be related to helping the patient control his life to reduce uncertainty and increase his independence. There are, however, very difficult circumstances such as the intensive care unit where the patient cannot feel either independent or in control. Staff should reduce anxiety, whether it is evident or not, by giving explanations before they do anything with a patient. One of the most orientating, stimulating events, which occurs to a semi-conscious or disoriented patient is the sound of a human voice. Such patients need to be told repeatedly where they are, what is happening and who they are with. A familiar friend or relative's voice is perhaps the best but Ashworth's (1978) paper on communications in an intensive care unit demonstrates a need and provides guidance for more verbal interaction to help these patients.

Trimble and Wilson-Barnett's (1974) paper for coronary care provides an introduction to preparing patients for psychological and physical recovery. Their recommendations follow others in this field which suggest a fore-warning of all likely events and feelings during recovery from a myocardial infarction. Anything which affects the patient's experience in the CCU and the ward should be explained before it happens. For example, before the patient stands or walks for the first time after two or three days of bed rest, possible feelings of weakness or dizziness should be anticipated and explained. If they do not occur, all to the good; if they do, however, the patient will not fear untoward complications of their coronary illness, as 'forewarned is forearmed'. Pamphlets from the National Heart Foundation can be useful but they are most useful for further illustration rather than an excuse for not giving any verbal account of what a heart attack is, what the effects are and how recovery can best be organised. Some hospitals organise a continuous programme of psychological support, where the nurse from the CCU is responsible for giving information, completing a care plan to that effect and providing several visits to the patient when he is on the ward. She also talks to and supports the spouse during the patient's recuperation in hospital. However, it is usually after discharge from hospital that questions and difficulties arise. A follow-up group for couples is, therefore, arranged two to four weeks after discharge, where staff discuss issues with patients and their partners and patients learn a great deal from each other.

SUPPORT FOR THE RELATIVES

The spouse or close relative of the patient is often more prone to worry than the patient himself. In the case of children this is particularly so. Nurses and doctors should be able to give information and up-to-date news of the patient's condition, even without being asked. If the relatives are kept informed and are consulted about treatments and plans, they will usually be far more helpful and relaxed while the patient is in hospital. Their appreciation and trust for the staff may also help to inspire the patient in this way too.

If the patient is very ill or if they are nursed in the intensive care unit, relatives may need extra support from the nurses. They can give them suggestions for relating to the patient, such as talking to the patient, despite an apparent lack of response, or just holding their hand. This seems very obvious but relatives are often over-awed by the complicated technology of the unit and frightened to do things in case they upset anything. Nurses can explain about the equipment to the relative and about the various drains and tubes. This may give the nurse the opportunity to get to know the relative but may also indicate that she cares enough about her patient to care about his relative too.

COMMUNICATIONS WITH OUT-PATIENTS

In the out-patients' clinic patients and their spouses should be given opportunities to relax sufficiently to ask questions and absorb information which the doctor or nurse wishes to give. From research discussed in Chapter 8, it seems evident that patients often suffer from a poor understanding of the doctor's communications. Ways for improving this situation are discussed by Ley and Spelman (1967). Although they refer specifically to the way a doctor should give information, it does, of course, apply to all staff who wish to share information and give explanation to their patients.

They stress that the patient's co-operation must be sought, not just assumed. Success in communication depends on the patient wanting to listen and understand. A team approach to care (involving patient, relative and staff) should, therefore, be sought. Information should be structured carefully, instructions should be given in a way that helps patients to understand their advantage. On no account should medical jargon be employed. It is also useful for patients to write things down, to be given the most important information first and for emphasis to be placed on the importance of instructions.

With specific reference to non-adherence to medications, Ley (1977) discussed ways for improving communications and thereby patient adherence to treatment. To increase patients' satisfaction, he suggests these stages:

1. Find out what worries the patient has.
2. Find out the patient's expectations.
3. Provide information about the diagnosis.
4. Adopt a friendly rather than business-like attitude.
5. Avoid medical jargon.
6. Spend time in conversation on non-medical topics.

Doctors and nurses should always ask for feedback on what they have told their patient as they can then gauge whether further explanation is necessary. Ley also recommends that in the patient–doctor interview it is advisable to first say what is wrong with the patient, then explain necessary treatment or tests and lastly stress

good listener, encourage conversation by repeating key words, making an effort to see the illness from the patient's point of view and accepting the patient as he conducts himself. As each person's psychological needs change from day to day, the nurse will need to accommodate her support and take a changing role which the patient assigns to her. The key to this advice is to be available when necessary and to act in accordance with the gravity of the situation.

THE GRIEVING PERSON

The ways in which staff can help the grieving person are remarkably similar to the methods advocated on pages 106 and 107 for helping the depressed patient. Staff should be aware of the important role they have to play in supporting bereaved relatives through the first stages of mourning. The most important thing, as Carlson (1970) says, is to prevent the grieving person from feeling alone or abandoned. When a relative visits a very sick or dying patient the nurses need to demonstrate their willingness to help by asking how the relative is, by asking if there is anything which might make visiting easier for them, etc. Later, when the patient dies, they should offer continuous support, perhaps by giving the ward telephone number or arranging for a community nurse to visit. Principles for supporting relatives include offering a sympathetic ear, allowing them to express their feelings and showing that you, as a staff member, care about their grief. Nurses and doctors should, of course, be aware of the heightened risk of physical and psychological illness during this time and should encourage a good diet and offer sedatives to help provide rest.

THE CRYING PATIENT

However, there are other difficulties which may inhibit the nurse's willingness and ability to communicate with their patient or their relative. People show their distress in many ways, and crying, which should convey a clear message for help, is often the most difficult expression of emotion to cope with for the staff. Robinson suggests that a nurse should sit or hand tissues while crying continues and not urge the patient to stop crying or to cheer up. Exploration of the reason for crying may begin when the patient has recovered. It is often difficult for a patient to explain why they are crying and this may infer to the patient that it is in some way less justified. They often feel 'it is silly to cry' and, therefore feel guilty about it. However, simply saying 'you must be feeling unhappy' in a kindly way may help the person to talk. If weeping is seen as an attempt to communicate, inexcusable habits of screening a patient and leaving them alone 'to get on with it' will hopefully disappear.

THE REGRESSED OR OVER-DEPENDENT PATIENT

In contrast to the patient who will not admit illness and who tries to do too much for himself, there are others who wish to abdicate responsibility for themselves and their recovery and continue in a passive patient role. This dependence becomes problematic when it extends beyond the period which is considered 'reasonable' by staff. A clear presentation of their expectations for the patient's behaviour and recovery throughout illness may help to prevent this.

If prolonged dependent behaviour occurs with apparent lack of motivation to help himself, the patient should receive well-considered care from staff. Reasons for this dependent behaviour may be discussed with some patients and it is often an unrealistic fear of lack of support in the future which hampers independence. Any attempts to help himself should be rewarded with praise and staff should encourage the patient by mentioning the advantages which accrue from more independence. Reassurance that help will be supplied in the future and discussion of what this will be should help to encourage the patient.

THE DEMANDING PATIENT

Many distressed patients have previously been labelled as demanding. Through lack of understanding about the patient's needs or feelings staff have covered their own inadequacies by ostracising and criticising the patient. The origin of demanding behaviour is often quite simply the patient's fears and lack of faith in the staff to help him. Because of his concern and anxiety for his condition he vents his feelings in a way which will provide him some attention and reassurance that he does matter. However, this behaviour tends to alienate him from the staff who realise their attempts to help do not give any satisfaction.

The solution to this situation is a firm resolution from a staff member to form a more trusting relationship with the patient in order to gain understanding of his worries and distress. This means that a nurse should go to the patient and sit down by him and try to talk to the patient about the situation. For example, she could say 'we don't seem to be very good at helping you, could you suggest if there is something else we might do?'. She might also start to go to the patient at times when she has not been summoned and simply chat to him. By indicating her concern it may be easier for the patient to communicate in a more understandable way.

Care of the aggressive patient is relevant to both general and psychiatric facilities. As Altschul (1971) says, 'aggressive behaviour can nearly always be traced to disturbances in the relationship between people'. It is usually a response to a frustrating or frightening experience.

In dealing with aggressive behaviour, the same principles of understanding and sympathy should be applied. Staff should attempt to realise why the patient felt aggressive. In discussing this, fears may be allayed and frustrating experiences prevented or modified.

FAILURE TO ACCEPT ILLNESS

Failure to accept illness (termed denial) through inability to cope with the threat and distress it would cause is also a major problem. Nurses and doctors cannot help the patient to adjust unless the patient himself accepts there is something wrong. As discussed in the previous Chapter, denial of illness is a generally non-adaptive defence against anxiety which may protect the patient initially, but in the long term may impede treatment. As Keining (1970) says, most people accept that management of this situation should not include attempts to break the denial, but staff should not endorse or collude in the denial. Their conversation should be reality orientated, giving truthful statements without arguing with the patient. Eventually denial usually gives way to a realistic depression and the patient can then be helped by the staff (Kubler Ross, 1969). If denial persists to the detriment of the patient's physical health it may be necessary to request a psychiatrist's assistance in coping with this reaction.

Mild forms of denial may be seen in many general hospital patients. For instance, talking humorously about their condition, denying its seriousness or talking about 'the old leg' as though it were not part of the patient, may be seen as a degree of 'denial'.

Refusal to accept illness and the role of patient may be seen in patients who display sexually oriented behaviour. This usually reflects a fear of severe illness or a denial of this because it threatens a person's sexuality. This occurs as a reaction against being dependent and obedient. Unfortunately, it often results in staff being frightened or even unkind to the patient. By understanding why this behaviour is used it should be possible to show the person that he is accepted and attractive and to make him feel more responsible and in control of his own life.

When coping with any of these problems it is essential to promote free communications among the staff. Recognition of the problem, clarification or interpretation should be discussed with all staff. Responsibility for nursing or medical intervention should only be planned after further understanding of the problem and talking to the patient. It is then usually advisable for one staff member to provide most of the psychological care. This avoids unnecessary repetition and lack of consistency in support given.

Doctors, social workers and nurses should discuss such psychological problems together. As shown previously gross disturbance in recovery may occur if depression 'sets in' or if unco-operative or over-demanding behaviour is allowed to cause a distance between staff and the patients. Goals for therapy should, therefore be explicit and assessed periodically by all who are involved in care.

As Robinson (1972) says, 'these formulations are only useful constructs. They are not valid truths but attempts to explain normal and aberrant behaviour'.

It is hoped that by discussing ways in which staff may be able to help patients they will feel more confident in approaching crying, angry, sexy or demanding patients. There is still so much opportunity for testing these approaches, but what we have established is the extensive need for this sort of therapy.

Bibliography

Abdellah, F. G. & Levine, E. (1965) *Better Patient Care through Nursing Research*. New York: Macmillan.

Abram, H. S. (1969) The Psychiatrist, the treatment of chronic renal failure and the prolongation of life. *American Journal of Psychiatry*, **126** (2), 157–67.

Abrams, R. D. (1974) *Not Alone with Cancer*. Illinois: Charles Thomas.

Aitken, R. C. B. & Zealley, A. K. (1970) Measurement of moods. *British Journal of Hospital Medicine*, **8**, 215–24.

Aitken-Swan, J. & Easson, E. (1959) Reactions of cancer patients on being told their diagnosis. *British Medical Journal*, **1**, 779.

Aitken-Swan, J. & Paterson, R. (1955) The cancer patient delay in seeking advice. *British Medical Journal*, **1**, 623.

Altschul, A. (1971) *Psychiatric Nursing*. 3rd edn. Nursing Aid Series. London: Bailliere, Tindall & Cassell.

Andrew, J. M. (1967) *Coping Styles, Stress-relevant Learning and Recovery from Surgery*. Ph. Dissertation Los Angeles: University of California.

Arnold, M. B. (1960) *Emotion and Personality*. Vol 1. Psychological Aspects. London: Cassell.

Ascione, F. & Ravin, R. (1975) Physician attitudes regarding patients' knowledge of prescribed medications. *Journal of the American Pharmaceutical Association*, **NS15**, 386–91.

Ashworth, P. (1978) Communication in the Intensive Care Unit. *Nursing Mirror*, **146**, (7), 34–6.

Ayd, F. J. (1961) *Recognising the Depressed Patient*. New York: Grune & Stratton.

Barnes, E. (1961) *People in Hospital*. London: Macmillan.

Bartemeir, L. H. (1961) Psychiatric aspects of medical practice. Emotional reactions to illness. *Maryland Medical Journal*, **10**, 240.

Bartrop, R. W., Lazarus, L., Luckhurst, E., Kiloh, L. G., & Penny, R. (1977) Depressed lymphocyte function after bereavement. *The Lancet*, **i**, 834–6.

Basovitz, H., Persk, H., Korchin, S. J. & Grinker, R. R. (1955) *Anxiety and Stress; an Interdisciplinary Study of a Life Situation*. London: McGraw Hill.

Baxter, S. (1975) Psychological problems of intensive care. *Nursing Times*, **71** (1), 22–3; **71** (2), 63–5.

Bellack, L. (Ed.) (1952) Psychology of Physical Illness. New York: Grune & Stratton.

Bennett, A. E., Garrod, J. & Halil, T. (1970) Chronic disease and disability in the community: a prevalence study. *British Medical Journal*, **3**, 762–4.

Bird, B. (1955) Psychological aspects of preoperative and postoperative care. *American Journal of Nursing*, **55** (6), 685–7.

Blackwell, B. (1976) Treatment adherence. *British Journal of Psychiatry*, **129**, 513–31.

Boore, J. R. P. (1976) An investigation into the effects of some aspects of preoperative preparation of patients on postoperative stress and recovery. *Ph.D. thesis*, University of Manchester.

Boore, J. R. P. (1977) Preoperative care of patients. *Nursing Times*, **73** (12), 409–11.

Brady, J. V. (1958) Ulcers in 'Executive' monkeys. Psychobiology. The Biological Bases of Behaviour. Readings from *The Scientific American*. San Francisco: Freeman.

Brewin, T. B. (1977) The cancer patient: communication and morale. *British Medical Journal*, **2**, 1623–7.

Brill, N. & Koegler, R. R. (1964) Controlled study of psychiatric out-patient treatment. *Archives of General Psychiatry*, **12**, 336–45.

Brocklehurst, J. C. & Shergold, M. (1968) What happens when geriatric patients leave hospital. *Lancet*, **ii**, 1133–5.

Brown, G. W. & Birley, J. L. T. (1968) Crises and life changes and the onset of schizophrenia. *Journal of Health and Social Behaviour*, **9**, 203.

Brown, G. W. (1975) *Guardian Newspaper Feature* 3rd April, 35.

Brown, J. R. (1950) Symposium on psychiatry and the general practitioner: the holistic treatment of neurologic disease. *Medical Clinics of North America*, **34**, 1019.

Byrne, D., Sternberg, M. A. & Schwartz, M. S. (1968) Relationship between depression sensitization and physical illness. *Journal of Abnormal Psychology*, **73**, 154–5.

Calhoun, J. B. (1962) Population density and social pathology. *Science Association*, **206** (2), 139–48.

Carlson, E. C. (Ed.) (1970) Grief and mourning. In *Behavioural Concepts and Nursing Intervention*. pp. 95–116. Philadelphia: Lippincott.

Carnevali, D. L. (1966) Pre-operative anxiety. *American Journal of Nursing*, **7**, 1536–8.

Carruthers, M. E. (1969) *The Lancet*, **ii**, 1170.

Cartwright, A. (1964) *Human Relations and Hospital Care* Institute of Community Studies. London: Routledge & Kegan Paul.

Cartwright, A., Hockey, L. & Anderson, J. L. (1973) *Life Before Death*. London: Routledge & Kegan Paul.

Cassel, J. (1974) Psychosocial processes and stress: theoretical formulation. *International Journal of Health Services*, **4**, (3), 471–82.

Castelnuovo-Tedescu, P. (1961) *Depression in Patients with Physical Disease*. New Jersey: Cranbury, Wallace Labs.

Cattell, R. B. (1972) in *Personality*. Ed. Lazarus, R. S. & Opton, E. M. Harmondsworth: Penguin.

Clarke, M. O. (1972) *An Aspect of Communication in the Health Service*. Unpublished Research Report.

Conger, J. J., Lawrey, W. & Turrell, E. S. (1958) The role of social experience in the production of gastric ulcers in rats placed in a conflict situation. *Journal of Abnormal and Social Psychology*, **57** (2), 214–20.

Coser, R. L. (1965) Some functions of laughter. In *Social Interaction and Patient Care*. Ed. Skipper, J. K. & Leonard, R. C. Philadelphia: Lippincott.

Davis, M. S. (1968) Variations in patients' compliance with doctors' advice: an empirical analysis of patterns of communication. *American Journal of Public Health*, **58**, 274–88.

Davitz, J. R. (1969) *The Language of Emotions*. New York: Academic Press.

Devlin, B. H., Plant, J. A. & Griffin, M. (1971) Aftermath of Surgery for Anorectal Cancer. *British Medical Journal*, **3**, 413.

De Wolfe, A. S., Barrell, R. P. & Cummings, J. W. (1966) Patient variables in emotional response to hospitalisation for physical illness. *Journal of Consulting Psychology*, **30**, (1), 68–72.

Egbert, L. D., Battit, G. E., Welch, C. E. & Bartlett, M. K. (1964) Reduction of post-operative pain by encouragement and instruction of patients. *New England Journal of Medicine*, **270**, 825-7.

Elms, R. R. & Leonard, R. C. (1966) Effects of nursing approaches during admission. *Nursing Research*, **15**, 39–48.

Endler, N. S., Hunt, McV. J. & Rosenstein, A. J. (1962) An S–R inventory of anxiousness. *Psychological Monographs*, 76. 17 No. 536.

Engel, G. L. (1962) *Psychological Development in Health and Disease*. Philadelphia: Saunders.

Engel, G. L. (1970) Conversion Symptoms. In *Signs and Symptoms*. Ed. MacBride, C. M. & Blacklow, R. S. pp. 650–68. Philadelphia: Lippincott.

Eysenck, H. J. & Eysenck, S. B. G. (1964)*Manual of the Eysenck Personality Inventory.* London: University of London Press.

Ferguson, T. (1961) Aftercare of the hospitalised patient. *British Medical Journal*, 1, 124–6.

Finnerty, F. M., Mattie, E. C. & Finnerty, F. A. (1973) Hypertension in the inner city. 1. Analysis of clinical drop-outs. *Circulation*, **XLVII**, 73–5.

Franklin, B. L. (1974)*Patient Anxiety on Admission to Hospital.* London: Rcn Study of Nursing Care Project.

Freedman, A. M., Kaplan, H. I. & Sadock, B. J. (1975)*Comprehensive Textbook of Psychiatry II.* Ch. 28. Baltimore: Williams & Wilkins.

French, K., Sutherland, E., Mitchell, H. & Mossman, S. (1977)*Study of patients' fears and worries.* Unpublished working paper.

Freud, A. (1939) *The Ego and Mechanisms of Defense.* New York: International University Press.

Friedman, S. B., Chodoff, P. & Mason, J. W. (1963) Behavioural observations on parents anticipating the death of a child. *Paediatrics*, 32, 610–25.

Friedman, E. A., Goodwin, N. J. & Chaudry, L. (1970) Psychosocial adjustment to maintenance haemodialysis. *New York State Journal of Medicine*, 70 (6), 767–74.

Garrity, T. F., Somes, G. W. & Marx, M. B. (1977) Personality factors in resistance to illness after recent life changes. *Journal of Psychosomatic Research*, 21, 23–32.

Glaser, B. & Strauss, A. (1965)*Awareness of Dying.* Chicago: Aldine Publishing Co.

Glaser, B. G. & Strauss, A. (1975) Dying in Hospital. In *Chronic Illness and the Quality of Life.* Ed. Strauss, A. New York: Mosby.

Glick, I. O., Weiss, R. S. & Parkes, C. M. (1974)*The First Year of Bereavement.* New York: Wiley-Interscience.

Goble, A. J., Adey, G. M. & Bullen, J. F. (1963) Rehabilitation of the coronary patient. *The Medical Journal of Australia*, 24, 975–82.

Goffman, E. (1961)*Asylums.* New York: Doubleday.

Goldman, J. & Schwab, J. J. (1965) Medical illness and patients' attitudes: somapsychic relationships. *Journal of Nervous and Mental Diseases*, 141 (6), 678.

Guinn, R. M. & Hill, H. (1964) Influence of anxiety on the relationship between self acceptance and acceptance of others. *Journal of Consulting Psychology*, 28, 116–19.

Hackett, T. P., Cassem, N. H. & Wishnie, H. A. (1968) The coronary care unit, an appraisal of its psychological hazards. *New England Journal of Medicine*, 278, 1365.

Hamilton, M. (1969) A diagnosis and rating of anxiety. In *Studies in Anxiety.* Ed. Lader, M. pp. 76–9. Ashford: Headly.

Hamilton Smith, S. (1971)*Nil by Mouth.* London: Rcn Study of Nursing Care Series.

Harvard, C. W. H. & Pearson, R. M. (1977) Use and effect of placebos. *Prescribers' Journal*, 4, 94–100.

Haynes, R. B. & Sackett, D. L. (1976) Compliance with Therapeutic Regimens, Appendix 1, 193–279. Maryland: Johns Hopkins University Press.

Hayward, J. (1975)*Information — A Prescription Against Pain.* London: Rcn Study of Nursing Care.

Hill, O. (1977) The psychological management of psychosomatic diseases. *British Journal of Psychiatry*, 131, 113–26.

Hoare, A. M. & Hawkins, C. F. (1976) Upper gastro-intestinal endoscopy with and without sedation: patients' opinions. *British Medical Journal*, 2, 20.

Hoch, P. H. & Zubin, H. (1950) *Anxiety.* New York: Grune & Stratton.

Hockey, L. (1966)*Feeling the Pulse: A Study of District Nursing in 6 Areas.* London: Queen's Institute of District Nursing.

Hockey, L. (1968)*Care in the Balance.* London: Queen's Institute of District Nursing.

Holmes, T. H. & Rahe, R. H. (1967) The social readjustment rating scale. *Journal of Psychosomatic Research*, 11, 213–18.

Hugh-Jones, P., Tanser, A. R. & Whitby, C. (1964) Patients view of admission to a London teaching hospital. *British Medical Journal*, 2, 660–4.

Imboden, J. B. (1972) Psychosocial determinants of recovery. *Advances in Psychosomatic Medicine*, 8, 142–55.

Izard, C. (1972)*Patterns of Emotions.* New York: Academic Press.

Janis, I. L. (1958) *Psychological Stress*. New York: Wiley.

Janis, I. L. & Mann, L. (1976) Coping with decisional conflict. *American Scientist*, **64**, 657–67.

Johnson, J. (1966) The influence of purposeful nurse–patient interaction on the patient's postoperative course. In *Exploring Progress in Medical-Surgical Nurse Practice*. pp. 16–22. American Nurses Association Monograph 2, New York.

Johnson, J. E. & Rice, V. H. (1974) Sensory and distress components of pain. *Nursing Research*, **23** (3), 203–8.

Johnson, J. E., Dabbs, J. M. & Leventhal, H. (1970) Psychosocial factors in the welfare of surgical patients. *Nursing Research*, **19** (1), 18–29.

Johnson, J. E., Kirchhoff, N. T. & Endress, M. P. (1975) Altering children's distress behaviour during orthopaedic cast removal. *Nursing Research*, **24** (6), 404–10.

Johnson, J. E., Morrissey, J. F. & Leventhal, H. (1973) Psychological preparation for an endoscopic examination. *Gastro-intestinal Endoscopy*, **19** (4), 180–2.

Joubert, P. & Lasagna, L. (1975) Patient package inserts. Nature, notions and needs. *Clinical Pharmacology and Therapeutics*, **18** (5), 507–13.

Joyce, C. (1962) Differences between physicians as revealed by clinical trials. *Proceedings of Royal Society of Medicine*, **55**, 776–8.

Kaplan de Nour, A. (1976) Psychotherapy with patients on chronic haemodialysis. *British Journal of Psychiatry*, **116** (531), 207–15.

Katz, J. L., Weiner, H. & Gallagher, T. F. (1970) Stress, distress and ego defenses. *Archives General Psychiatry*, **23**, 131–4.

Keining, M. M. (1970) Denial of illness. In *Behavioural Concepts and Nursing Intervention*. Ed. Carlson, E.C. Philadelphia: Lippincott.

Kielholz, P. (Ed.) (1973) *Masked Depression*. Vienna: Huber.

Koos, E. (1954) *The Health of Regionsville: What the People Thought and Did About It*. New York: Columbia University Press.

Kronfield, D. S. (1969) Psychiatric view of the intensive care unit. *British Medical Journal*, **1**, 108–10.

Korsch, B. and Negrete, V. (1972) Doctor-patient communication. *Scientific American*, **227**, 66.

Kubler Ross, E. (1969) *On Death and Dying*. New York: Macmillan.

Lader, M. & Marks, I. (1971) *Clinical Anxiety*. London: Heinemann.

Langer, E. J., Janis, I. L. & Wolfer, J. A. (1975) Reduction of psychological stress in surgical patients. *Journal of Experimental and Social Psychology*, **11**, 155–65.

Langer, T. & Michaels, S. (1963) *Life Stress and Mental Health*. London: Glencoe Free Press.

Lazarus, R. S. (1966) *Psychosocial Stress and the Coping Process*. New York: McGraw Hill.

Lazarus, R. S. (1967) Cognitive and Personality Factors Underlying Threat and Coping. In *Psychological Stress*. Ed. Appley, M. & Trumbul, R. New York: Appleton Century Croft.

Lazarus, H. R. & Hagans, J. H. (1968) Prevention of psychosis following open heart surgery. *American Journal of Psychiatry*, **124** (9), 1190–5.

Leigh, J. M., Walker, J. & Janaganathan, P. (1977) Effect of pre-operative anaesthetic visit on anxiety. *British Medical Journal*, **2**, 987–9.

Levitt, E. E. (1971) *The Psychology of Anxiety*. London: Granada Publishing.

Levitt, R. (1974) Becoming a patient. *Community Health*, **6**, 138–41.

Levitt, R. (1975) Attitudes of hospital patients. *Nursing Times*, **71** (13), 497–9.

Levy, N. B. & Wynbrandt, G. D. (1975) The Quality of Life on Maintenance Haemodialysis. *Lancet*, **1**, 1328–30.

Ley, P. (1977) Patient compliance – a psychologist's viewpoint. *Prescribers' Journal*, **17**, 1.

Ley, P. & Spelman, M. (1967) *Communicating with the Patient*. St. Albans: Staples Press.

Ley, P., Bradshaw, P. W. & Eaves, D. (1973) A method for increasing patients' recollection of information presented by doctors. *Psychological Medicine*, **3**, 217–20.

Liddell, H. (1950) Some Specific Factors that Modify Tolerance for Environmental

Stress. In *Life Stress and Bodily Disease*. Wolff, H. G., Wolff, S. G. & Hare, C. C. pp. 155–71. Baltimore: Williams and Williams.

Lindeman, C. A. & Van Aernam, B. (1971) Nursing intervention with the pre-surgical patient – The effects of structured and unstructured pre-operative teaching. *Nursing Research*, **20**, 319–32.

Lindeman, E. (1944) Symptomatology and management of acute grief. *American Journal of Psychiatry*, **101**, 7–21.

Lipowski, Z. J. (1967) Review of consultation psychiatry and psychosomatic medicine, 2. Clinical aspects. *Psychosomatic Medicine*, **29** (3), 201–24.

Lipowski, Z. J. (1975) Physical illness, the patient and his environment: psychosocial foundations of medicine. *American Handbook of Psychiatry*, Vol 4, 1–42.

Lishman, A. (1972) Selective factors in memory, Part 2 affective disorders. *Psychological Medicine*, **2**, 248–53.

Lloyd, G. G. (1977) Psychological reactions of physical illness. *British Journal of Hospital Medicine*, **2**, 352–8.

Lucente, F. E. & Fleck, S. (1972) A study of hospitalisation anxiety in 408 medical and surgical patients. *Psychosomatic Medicine*, **34** (4), 304–11.

Lynn, R. (1971) *National Differences in Anxiety*. London: The Economic and Social Research Institute. Monograph 2.

Maguire, G. P. (1975) The psychological and social consequences of breast cancer. *Nursing Mirror*, **140** (14), 53–5.

Maguire, G. P. (1976) The Psychological & Social Sequelae of Mastectomy. In *Modern Perspectives in Psychiatric Aspects of Surgery*. Ed. Howells, J. New York: Bruner Macel.

Maguire, G. P. (1978) The Psychological Effects of Cancers and their Treatments. In *Oncology for Nurses*. Vol 2. Ed. Tiffany, B. London: Allen & Unwin.

Marston, M. V. (1970) Compliance with medical regimens: a review of the literature. *Nursing Research*, **19** (4), 313–32.

Matthews, D. (1975) The non-compliant patient. *Primary Care*, **2** (2), 284–94.

May, R. (1950) *The Meaning of Fear*. New York: Ronald Press.

McGhee, A. (1961) *The Patient's Attitude to Nursing Care*. Edinburgh: Livingstone.

McIntosh, J. (1976) Patients' awareness and desire for information about undisclosed malignant disease. *Lancet*, **2**, 300.

Mechanic, D. (1962) The concept of illness behaviour. *Journal of Chronic Diseases*, **15**, 189–94.

Melia, K. M. (1977) The intensive care unit – a stress situation. *The Nursing Times*, **73** (5), 17–20.

Merskey, H. & Trimble, M. R. (1979) Personality and other factors promoting conversion symptoms. *American Journal of Psychiatry*, **136** (2), 179–182.

Meyers, M. E. (1964) The effects of types of communication on patients' reactions to stress. *Nursing Research*, **13** (2), 126–31.

Minckley, B. B. (1974) Physiological and psychological responses of elective surgical patients. *Nursing Research*, **23** (5), 392–401.

Moffic, H. S. & Paykel, E. S. (1975) Depression in medical in-patients. *British Journal of Psychiatry*, **126**, 346–53.

Moran, P. (1963) *Unpublished Thesis* Yale University (quoted by Janis, I. (1971) In *Stress and Frustration*. New York: Harcourt Brace).

Nagle, R., Gangola, R. & Picton Robinson, I. (1971) Factors influencing return to work after myocardial infarction. *Lancet*, **ii**, 454–6.

Neary, D. (1976) Neuropsychiatric sequelae of renal failure. *British Medical Journal*, **1**, 122–30.

Nuckalls, C. B., Cassel, J. & Kaplan, B. H. (1972) Psychosocial assets, life crises and the prognosis of pregnancy. *American Journal Epidemiology*, **95**, 431–44.

Oken, D. (1961) What to tell cancer patients: a study of medical attitudes. *Journal of American Medical Association*, **175**, 1120–8.

Olmsted, R. W. & Kennedy, D. A. (1975) In *Medical Behavioural Science*. Ed. Millon, T. pp. 200–6. London: Saunders.

Park, L. & Covi, L. (1965) Non-blind placebo trial. *Archives of General Psychiatry*, 12, 336–45.

Parkes, C. M. (1972) Components of the reaction to loss of a limb, spouse or home. *Journal of Psychosomatic Research*, 16, 343–9.

Parkes, C. M., Benjamin, B. & Fitzgerald, R. G. (1969) Broken heart: a statistical study of increased mortality among widowers. *British Medical Journal*, 1, 740–3.

Parsons, T. (1951) *The Social System*. Illinois: Glencoe Free Press.

Paykel, E. S. (1974) Life stress and psychiatric disorder. In *Stressful Life Events: Their Nature and Effects*. Ed. Dohrenwend, B. S. & Dohrenwend, B. P. pp. 135–9. New York: Wiley.

Paykel, E. S., Klerman, G. L. & Prusoff, B. A. (1976) Personality and symptom pattern in depression. *British Journal of Psychiatry*, 129, 327–34.

Penrose, R. J. J. (1972) Life events before subarachnoid haemorrhage. *Journal of Psychosomatic Research*, 16, 329–33.

Pilowsky, I. (1975) Dimensions of abnormal illness behaviour. *Australian & New Zealand Journal of Psychiatry*, 9, 141–7.

Porter, A. M. W. (1969) Drug defaulting in a general practice. *British Medical Journal*, 1, 18–22.

Rachman, S. J. & Philips, C. (1975) *Psychology and Medicine*. London: Temple Smith.

Rahe, R. H. (1968) Life-change measurement as a predictor of illness. *Proceedings of the Royal Society of Medicine*, 1121, 8.

Rahe, R. H. (1975) A liaison psychiatrist on the coronary care unit. In *Consultation—Liaison Psychiatry*. Ed. Pasnau, R. O. Ch. 8. New York: Grune & Stratton.

Rahe, R. H., McKean, D. J. & Arthur, R. J. (1967) A longitudinal study of life-change and illness patterns. *Journal of Psychosomatic Research*, 10, 335–66.

Raphael, W. (1969) *Patients and their Hospitals*. King Edward Fund for London.

Rees, L. W. (1976) Stress, Distress and Disease. *British Journal of Psychiatry*, 128, 3–18.

Roberts, I. (1975) *Discharged from Hospital*. London: Rcn Study of Nursing Care Research Project.

Robinson, L. (1972) *Psychological Aspects of the Care of Hospitalised Patients*, 3rd edn. Philadelphia: Davis.

Roger, B. (1975) The role of the psychiatrist in the renal dialysis unit. In *Consultation—Liaison Psychiatry*. Ed. Pasnau, R. O. Ch. 11. New York: Grune & Stratton.

Rosenberg, M. (1962) The association between self-esteem and anxiety. *Journal of Psychiatric Research*, 6, 135–51.

Rosenman, R. H. (1976) Paper at the *Annual Meeting of the Society for Psychosomatic Research*, London.

Roth, H. P. & Berger, D. G. (1960) Studies on patient cooperation in ulcer treatment observation of actual as compared to prescribed antacid intake on a hospital ward. *Gastroenterology*, Apx. 38, 630–3.

Ruff, G. E. & Korchin, S. J. (1967) Adaptive stress behaviour. In *Psychological Stress*. Ed. Appley, M. & Trumbul, R. New York: Appleton Century Croft.

Rycroft, C. (1968) *Anxiety and Neurosis*. London: Pelican.

Sainsbury, P. (1973) A comparative evaluation of a comprehensive community psychiatric service. In *Policy for Action: A Comparative Evaluation of a Community Psychiatric Service*. Ed. Cawley, R. & McLachlan, G. pp. 129–43. London: Oxford University Press.

Sarnoff, I. & Zimbardo, P. G. (1961) Anxiety, fear and social affiliation. *Journal of Abnormal and Social Psychology*, 62, 356–63.

Saunders, C. (1976) In *Scientific Foundations of Oncology*. Ed. Symington, T. London: Heinemann.

Schachter, S. (1959) *The Psychology of Affiliation*. California: Stanford University Press.

Schwab, J. (1968) *Handbook of Psychiatric Consultation*. pp. 189–95. New York: Appleton Century Croft.

Schwab, J. J., Bidlow, M., Brown, J. M. & Holzer, C. E. (1967) Diagnosing depression in medical in-patients. *Annals of Internal Medicine*, 67 (4), 695–706.

Scotch, N. A. (1960) Sociocultural factors in the epidemiology of Zulu hypertension. *American Journal of Public Health*, 53, 1205–13.

Selye, H. (1956) *The Stress of Life*. New York: McGraw-Hill.

Selye, H. (1973) The evolution of the stress concept. *American Scientist*, 61, 692–9.

Senescu, R. A. (1963) The development of emotional complications in the patient with cancer. *Journal of Chronic Diseases*, 16, 813.

Shapiro, A. K., Streuning, E. L., Barten, H. & Shapiro, E. (1975) Correlates of placebo reaction in an outpatient population. *Psychological Medicine*, 5, 389–96.

Shneidman, E. S. (1975) Postvention the care of the bereaved. In *Consultation—Liaison Psychiatry*. Ed. Pasnau, R. O. New York: Grune & Stratton.

Skeet, M. (1970) *Home From Hospital*. London: The Dan Mason Nursing Research Committee.

Smith, E. A. (1976) *Psychosocial Aspects of Cancer Patient Care*. New York: McGraw Hill.

Spielberger, C. D. (1972) *Anxiety, Current Trends in Theory and Research*, Vol. 1. London: Academic Press.

Spitz, R. A. (1946) Anaclitic depression. *Psychoanalytic Study of Child*, 2, 313–42.

Stacey, M. (1970) *Hospitals, Children and their Families*. London: Routledge & Kegan Paul.

Starrett, D. (1961) Psychiatric mechanisms in severe disability. *Rocky Mountain Medical Journal*, 58, 42.

Stephenson, C. A. (1977) Stress in critically ill patients. *American Journal of Nursing*, 11, 1806–9.

Stockwell, F. (1972) *The Unpopular Patient*. London: Rcn Study of Nursing Care Series.

Strauss, A. (1975) *Chronic Illness and the Quality of Life*. New York: C. V. Mosby Co.

Sullivan, H. S. (1956) *Clinical Studies in Psychiatry*. New York: Norton.

Summers, D. H. (1978) Ch. 9 Care of the dying. In *Oncology for Nurses*. Ed. Tiffany, B. London: Allen & Unwin.

Swift, N. I. (1962) Psychological reactions to illness. *Physiotherapy*, 48, 172.

Taylor, D. A., Wheeler, L. & Altman, F. (1968) Stress relations in socially isolated groups. *Journal of Personality and Social Psychology*, 9, 369–76.

Thiel, H. G., Parker, D. & Bruce, T. A. (1973) Stress factors and the risk of myocardial infarction. *Journal of Psychosomatic Research*, 17, 43–57.

Thompson, M. R. (1978) Ch. 2 Communication with patients and relatives. In *Oncology for Nurses*. Ed. Tiffany, B. London: Allen & Unwin.

Titchener, J. L. & Levine, M. (1960) Surgery as a Human Experience: *The Psychodynamics of Surgical Practice*. New York: Oxford University Press.

Trimble, M. & Wilson-Barnett, J. (1974) Psychological needs of coronary patients. *Nursing Times*, 70 (38), 1464–5.

Uhlenhuth, E. H. & Paykel, E. S. (1973) Symptom configuration and life events. *Archives General Psychiatry*, 28, 744–8.

Vetter, N. J., Cay, E. L., Phillip, A. E. & Strange, R. G. (1977) Anxiety on admission to a coronary care unit. *Journal of Psychosomatic Research*, 21, 73–8.

Volicer, B. J. & Bohannon, M. W. (1973) Perceived stress levels of events associated with the experience of hospitalisation. *Nursing Research*, 32, (6), 491–7.

Watkins, J. D., Roberts, D. E., Williams, T. F., Martin, D. A. & Coyle, V. (1967) Observation of medication errors made by diabetic patients in the home. *Diabetes*, 16, (12), 882–5.

Weisman, A. D. (1975) The dying patient. In *Consultation—Liaison Psychiatry*. Ed. Pasnau, R. O. New York: Grune & Stratton.

Welgram, P. R. (1974) Learned control of gastric acid secretion in ulcer patients. *Psychosomatic Medicine*, 26, 411–19.

Wild, A. A. & Evans, J. (1968) The patient and the X-ray department. *British Medical Journal*, 3, 107–9.

Wilson-Barnett, J. (1976) Patients' emotional reactions to hospitalization: an exploratory study. *Journal of Advanced Nursing*, **1**, 351–8.

Wilson-Barnett, J. (1977) *Patients' Emotional Reactions to Hospitalisation*. Ph.D. Thesis, University of London.

Wilson-Barnett, J. (1978) In hospital patients' feelings and opinions. *Nursing Times* Occasional Papers, **74** (8), 29–32.

Wilson-Barnett, J. (1978) Patients' emotional responses to barium X-rays. *Journal of Advanced Nursing*, **3** (1), 37–46.

Wilson-Barnett, J. & Carrigy, A. (1978) Factors affecting patients' responses to hospitalisation. *Journal of Advanced Nursing*, **3** (3), 221–8.

Wishnie, H. A., Hackett, T. P. & Cassem, N. H. (1971) Psychological hazards of convalescence following myocardial infarction. *Journal of American Medical Association*, **215** (8), 1292–6.

Wrigglesworth, J. M. & Williams, J. T. (1975) The construction of an objective test to measure patient satisfaction. *International Journal of Nursing Studies*, **12**, 123–32.

Wynn, A. (1967) Unwarranted emotional distress in men with ischaemic heart disease. *Medical Journal of Australia*, **2**, 847.

Yalom, I. D. & Greaves, C. (1977) Group therapy with the terminally ill. *American Journal of Psychiatry*, **134**, 396–400.

Author Index

Subject Index

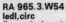
DATE DUE

RETURNED

OCT 2 6 1992

RETURNED

RETURNED

RETURNED

RETURNED

SEP 1 5 1998

NOV 1 5 2005